All Diabetes therapy concepts and solutions

Contents

Disclaimer
Copyright
Introduction
All Diabetes therapy concepts and solutions
   Type 1 diabetes and celiac disease...
What happens in the small intestine with the manifestation of celiac disease?
   What symptoms indicate celiac disease?
What is the difficulty with the gluten-free diet?
Knowledge refreshed What is gluten?
Children and adolescents with type 1: eat like everyone else?
Three Rules
   And what do children with diabetes eat?
Training
   Who is being trained?
   What is being trained?
   What is the training done with?
Intensive therapy: imitate nature!
Healthy diet & reasonable weight - With insulin therapy: break weight gain!
Losing weight successfully: the first steps Check your eating habits.
   Helps!
   Running, cycling, hiking: all good for you!
Too much insulin? Check more often!
   Is fasting a Solution?
All about insulin
   Short-acting human insulins
   Lente insulins
   Long-acting insulin
   Genetic engineering: side effects?

Diabetes and smoking: ominous!
- Even passive smoking: dangerous!
- But how to stop?
- Behavioral therapy: Avoid cigarette smoke!

Type 2 diabetes – or rather "insulin resistance disease"
- Conclusion

Type 2 diabetes and hypertension: from expert opinion to evidence
- Are there other cardiovascular risk factors?
- Conclusion
- Exciting result

Drug therapy
- Summary

Hypoglycemia problems in diabetes mellitus – Etiology, diagnostics, and treatment
- Introduction
- Self-management and hypoglycemia problems

Diagnostic

Running in comparison with heavy physical exertion for the prevention of cardiovascular events in women
- Methods:
- Results:
- Conclusion:
- Comment:
- "Fat burner" sports
- Swimming
- Walking and Nordic Walking
- Cycling

Eating disorders: consultants and doctors are important mediators
- Slimming mania as a cause?
- Diagnostic criteria
- Diagnostic criteria
- Conclusion

Relatives – (not) a topic?! - Mastering diabetes together
Diabetes and Depression – Coping with Depression and Diabetes
The Future of Diabetes Treatment: Is a Cure Possible? Yes, CLICK HERE

Disclaimer

The information contained in this book, or on websites linked from this book, is for education purposes only and is not a substitute for medical advice from a doctor or health care provider. Consult a health care provider for advice about any course of treatment, medical condition, or before marking any changes to diet or exercise.

The Future of Diabetes Treatment: Is a Cure Possible? Yes, CLICK HERE

Copyright

Copyright © 2021 A.W. Ansari. All rights reserved. Including the right to reproduce this book or portions thereof, in any form. No part of this text may be reproduced in any form without the express written permission of the author. Version 2021.07.06

Introduction

If you're trying to get a realistic understanding of this disease, what you need to keep yourself healthy, and how to cope with the many social and psychological challenges of diabetes, it may not be so obvious which books are right for you. I've been publishing diabetes books for many years. People often ask us about the best books for type 1 diabetes and the best books for type 2 diabetes... but our view is that there is enough commonality that most books apply well to both. Get you started on your "best-of" diabetes reading.

The Future of Diabetes Treatment: Is a Cure Possible? Yes, CLICK HERE

All Diabetes therapy concepts and solutions

Type 1 diabetes and celiac disease...

what to do if both diseases occur together type 1 diabetes and celiac disease are two completely different diseases. Nevertheless, there are increasing reports of an increased incidence of celiac disease in people with type 1 diabetes. This places special demands on the therapy and training of those affected. Definitions of terms Celiac disease/sprue:

Celiac disease: Child form of gluten-sensitive enteropathy

Sprue: An adult form of gluten-sensitive enteropathy.

Both forms lead to characteristic inflammatory damage to the small intestine with the loss of intestinal villi.

Celiac disease and type 1 diabetes – what do they have to do with each other?

Celiac disease (synonym: gluten-sensitive enteropathy or native sprue) is a disease of the small intestine that leads to atrophy of the small intestine in genetically predisposed people through an immunologically abnormal reaction to components of the cereal protein (gluten) and thus to a malabsorption syndrome. Through a life-long strictly gluten-free diet, successful treatment is possible.

Even in type 1 diabetes, autoimmune reactions lead to a symptom-inducing absolute insulin deficiency. The subsequent dysregulation of glucose metabolism is compensated by insulin treatment and a targeted carbohydrate intake. Bans on food choice no longer exist today.

Despite the differences between the two diseases, there are connections, and there are people who have both diseases at the same time.

While only 0.3 to 0.5% of the normal population have celiac disease, this figure is significantly higher in type 1 diabetics, namely

5 to 7%.

In diabetes centers, freshly manifested type 1 diabetics are therefore examined for celiac antibodies. Celiac, on the other hand, have a lower risk of developing type 1 diabetes the longer they eat a gluten-free diet. In the combination of type 1 diabetes and celiac disease, diabetes usually occurs first. Genetic predisposition is the prerequisite for the development of both diseases. In type 1 diabetes, there is a close relationship to genes of the immune system: For example, B HLA-DR3 and/or HLA-DR4 genes occur in about 90% of patients with type 1 diabetes, but only in 40-50% of the normal population. Celiac disease/sprue also has a connection to genes in the HLA region: the antigens HLA-DQ2 and HLA-DQ8 occur in 80-90% of celiac patients.

	Type 1 diabetes	Celiac disease/sprue
Detection of autoimmune disease	- Islet cell antibodies (ICA)	- Endomysium antibodies (EMA)
	- Gliadin decarboxylase antibodies (GAD)	- Anti-gliadin antibodies
	- Tyrosine phosphatase	- IgA antibodies against tissue transglutaminase
	IA-2A and IA-2ß	
	- Insulin autoantibodies (IAA)	

frequency	About 0.3% of the population, i.e. 1:300	Approx. 0.15% - 0.3% of the population, i.e. 1:150 to 1:300
genetics	HLA-DR3 and/or HLA-DR4 in approximately 90% of patients	HLA-DQ2 and HLA-DQ8 in 80-90% of patients
Factors of origin	Exogenous triggers are suspected, z.B. - Viral infections - Vaccinations - Diet (gluten-containing?)	Gluten/gliadin and related cereal proteins as a triggering agent
therapy	insulin The autoimmunological	Gluten-free diet In compliance with the

	destruction of the insulin-	gluten-free diet, there is
	forming cells in the	extensive regeneration of
	the pancreas is irreversible, i.e.	the small intestinal
	the insulin deficiency	mucosa
	remains for life	

What happens in the small intestine with the manifestation of celiac disease?

The surface of the small intestine is enlarged by folds and protrusions so that the absorption of the nutrients can take place optimally. With an intolerance of gluten, a normal (i.e. gluten-containing) diet leads to damage to the small intestine. Due to the contact of gluten with the cells of the intestinal mucosa, the characteristic changes of the small intestine epithelium with loss of intestinal villi arise. In this process, the surface area of the intestine is reduced in size and not enough nutrients can be absorbed (malabsorption syndrome). The non-absorbed food components can lead to diarrhea and flatulence.

What symptoms indicate celiac disease?

In the clinical symptoms of celiac disease, a distinction is made between intestinal and extra-intestinal symptoms (see Table 2).

Intestinal symptoms	Extra intestinal manifestations
- Diarrhea	- Anemia
- Meteorism	- Hair loss

- Weight loss	- Bleeding
- Mouth angle and tongue changes	- Osteopenia, osteoporosis
	- Muscle atrophy
	- Peripheral neuropathy
	- Amenorrhea, infertility, impotence
	- Hyperkeratosis
	- Dermatitis
	- Tooth damage
	- Edema

Celiac disease does not always show up with the classic intestinal symptoms such as diarrhea, foul-smelling flatulence, and vomiting. Sprue often contains only mildly pronounced or atypical forms associated with anemia due. B to iron deficiency, osteoporosis due to calcium and vitamin D deficiency, joint complaints, bone pain, pale skin, tooth damage, or low neurological symptoms. Celiac disease is only partly noticeable due to secondary lactose intolerance, which leads to corresponding intestinal symptomatology.

The clinically symptom-free celiac disease must also be treated, as it can have significant consequences. Malignant small intestine lymphomas, other autoimmune diseases (including type 1 diabetes and thyroid diseases), and dermatitis herpetiformis occur much more frequently in unrecognized and untreated celiac patients than in treated patients. A gluten-free diet seems to largely prevent these diseases associated with sprue.

What causes the damage to the small intestinal mucosa in the metabolism of type 1 diabetic?

In patients with pre-existing type 1 diabetes, hypoglycemia often occurs in the active disease phase of celiac disease as a result of malabsorption.

Despite the constant dose of insulin, the carbohydrate intake must be reduced.

In the case of untreated celiac disease, the small intestinal mucosa is so damaged that even the carbohydrates are not absorbed properly. Treatment with gluten-free nutrition leads to the regeneration of the small intestinal mucosa and the normalization of insulin requirements. The number of hypoglycemia decreases, the metabolic situation stabilizes.

The therapy for celiac disease/sprue means gluten-free diet Celiac disease, like diabetes, is a chronic disease and cannot be treated medicinally, but only by a strictly gluten-free diet.

Diet in celiac disease means the abandonment of all gluten-containing cereals such as wheat (spelled, green kernel), rye, barley, and oats. All foods that contain these cereals must be consistently avoided. The toxic effect of the evening in oats is not assured; there is evidence that oats are tolerated in quantities up to 50 grams per day. However, oats should also be eliminated in the initial phase of treatment. In the case of processed foods that are not prepared by the authorities, gluten must always be added. The correct selection of gluten-free foods is possible based on the "List of gluten-free foods", which the German Celiac Society publishes annually (see the end of text). Without this list, a gluten-free diet is difficult. For cereal products to be avoided, there are numerous gluten-free substitute products. Gluten-free raw materials for the production of baked and pasta are in particular corn, rice, buckwheat, millet, soy, and potato flour.

However, gluten-free finished products are mostly made of starch, so they have a high glycemic index. This must be taken into account with appropriate insulin therapy (e.B. with rapidly effective insulin analogs). For this reason, intensified insulin therapy is the treatment of choice. The production of gluten-free bread from millet, buckwheat, whole rice, corn, and soy is a suitable way to reduce the postprandial increase in blood sugar. In the severe form with diarrhea and steatorrhea (malabsorption), MCT fats and water-soluble fiber should be given.

In the case of simultaneous lactose intolerance, lactose-containing foods should also be avoided. Therefore, the consultation should in any case be provided by a nutritionist (dietician, graduate Anthropologie).

Gluten-free foods Meat, fish, eggs, natural dairy products, natural cheeses (caution: mold cheese), butter, margarine, oils, potatoes, legumes (also soy), fresh vegetables and fruits, sugar, honey, jams, herbs, salt, corn, rice, millet, quinoa, amaranth, buckwheat, nuts, sesame, sunflower and pumpkin seeds, poppies, flaxseed, pure cocoa, mineral water, pure fruit juices, coffee, non-flavored tea, wine, sparkling wine, brandy.

Gluten-containing foods wheat, spelled, green kernel, rye, barley, oats, wild rice in all forms of condition (flour, semolina, barley, germs, bran, meal, flakes), bread, baked goods, pasta, cereals, many ready meals, cereal coffee, beer.

Possibly gluten-containing foods (depending on the manufacturer) vegetable and fruit preparations, dairy products with fruit preparation, cheese preparations, dried fruits, fish products, spice mixtures, mustard, ketchup, condiments, vinegar, binders, curing aids, cutter aids, French fries, mashed potatoes, chips, light products, popcorn, confectionery, flavored tea, fruit juice drinks, liqueurs, whiskey and much more.

What is the difficulty with the gluten-free diet?

Gluten is not subject to declaration, i.e. it does not have to be indicated as gluten on the list of ingredients of the packaging of food!

There are ready-to-eat foods that consist of several ingredients. Example: yogurt with fruit preparation. The ingredients for fruit preparation do not have to be indicated if they do not exceed a quarter of the quantity of the total product. This is where gluten can hide. If the components of the compound ingredient are less than 25% of the total product, they do not have to be declared.

A varied, gluten-free diet is possible with the help of the "List of gluten-free foods" of the German Celiac Society.

Knowledge refreshed What is gluten?

Gluten is a protein component of the cereals wheat, rye, oats, barley, spelled and green kernel. The cereal protein is localized in the endosperm of the grain and consists of many protein fractions. Wheat, for example, has a protein content of 7 to 15%, which consists of 90% gluten. Gluten can be divided into proclamation and glutenin. The disease-causing effect is the polyamines (= alcohol-soluble fraction of gluten). The protamines are named differently in different cereals:

Cerea:	Proclamation:
Wheat	Gliadin
Rye	Saline
Barley	Horde in
Oats	A venin

The cause of the intolerance lies in an antigen-antibody reaction of the body against these polypeptides. The Dutch researchers Dicke, Weijers, and van den Kamer only recognized gluten in the years 1950-1953 as a damaging in the development of celiac disease. Gluten has fantastic properties as a functional protein: it gels, it emulsifies, it stabilizes. Gluten can also hide behind the term "technological excipient" in processed foods.

Conclusion

For celiac, a gluten-free diet is the only possible therapy.

The banishment of the disease-causing agent can lead to the complete regeneration of the intestinal mucosa. If type 1 diabetes is already present, it is important to take into account the high glycemic index of gluten-free carbohydrates and to compensate with the means of intensified insulin therapy.

Caring for a type 1 diabetic with celiac disease presents a real challenge for any therapist, which will be ineffective without being led to self-management. Both diseases in combination can only be treated satisfactorily if the patient learns to bear the responsibility himself.

Due to the known associations of both diseases with other autoimmune diseases, future studies will have to show whether a gluten-free diet can also play a role in the primary prevention of type 1 diabetes mellitus

Children and adolescents with type 1: eat like everyone else?

Insulin therapy is an important pillar in the treatment of type 1 diabetics. Another is how those affected eat and drink. How should type 1 diabetics eat and how can this content be conveyed by the treatment team? These questions are answered by diabetes professional author Maike Grotzke.

For children and adolescents with type 1 diabetes, we recommend, like all other children, a healthy, varied, full-fledged mixed diet. This can be implemented practicable, e.B. with the "Optimized Mixed Diet", called "OptimiX" for short, of the Dortmund Research Institute for Child Nutrition (FKE). "Optimus" is based on the current recommendations for nutrient intake (DACH 2000). It takes into account medical aspects of the prevention of nutritionally affected diseases, e.B. cardiovascular diseases, caries, or obesity. When choosing food, no special foods or diet products are recommended, but commercially available, inexpensive products. Furthermore, preferences for sweets, fried foods, or fast food can be taken into account, since a proportion of the calorie intake for "tolerated foods" is planned into the "optimized mixed food". Dietary habits of three main meals (two bread meals and a hot meal) and two to three intermediate meals (a school breakfast, a vesper, a late meal, or another school breakfast) are well compatible with these recommendations.

Accept eating behavior The recommendations for energy intake are intended as a guide and apply to averagely active children and adolescents.

They must be individually adapted e.B. in case of overweight or underweight. Practical experience shows that in most cases the spontaneous eating behavior of the children corresponds to their physiological energy requirements. For this reason, it makes no sense to intervene in the eating behavior of children and to want to regulate it. This means, however, that the daily amounts of insulin must be adapted to the eating behavior of children and adolescents 10 to 20 % proteins The recommended protein requirement is 2.0 g/kg BW (body weight) for infants and 0.9 g/kg BW for adolescents.

In a teenager, this corresponds to a daily amount of protein of about 50 grams. In total, 10 – 20% of the total energy is to be covered by proteins.

Not too much fat The fat intake should – except infant and young children nutrition – not exceed 35% of the total energy.

To achieve a healthy fat selection, to reduce saturated fatty acids and increase the intake of unsaturated fatty acids, vegetable fats should preferably be eaten. In particular, soybean, corn germ, rapeseed, or olive oil should be mentioned here. Due to their negative effect, trans fatty acids should be reduced e.B. to the increase of LDL cholesterol and lowering HDL cholesterol in the daily diet. Trans fatty acids are hydrogenated fats that are predominantly found in finished products, puff pastries, potato chips, or chocolate.

Many carbohydrates and fiber The carbohydrate content should be at least 50% of the total energy, as in metabolically healthy children and adolescents.

With "OptimiX" this is usually easy to realize because plenty of plant-based foods are recommended. Here, the emphasis should be placed on carbohydrates with a low glycemic index, e.B. whole grains, fruits, and vegetables. Children's preference for sweet foods or sweets can also be taken into account with a desired moderate intake of sucrose and incorporated into the daily diet. The recommendation is a maximum of 10% of the total energy. These are usually two to three BE/KE daily, which corresponds to e.B a chocolate bar or a piece of cake. For the daily fiber intake, there are no guideline values for children. However, an amount of 10 grams per 1000 calories seems feasible. For a 12-year-old child, this would be an amount of about 20 grams of fiber daily. If a child eats two slices of multi-grain bread, a portion of cereal, a piece of fruit, and two portions of vegetables a day, he has eaten the required amount of 20 grams of fiber. This recommendation is initially very theoretical and difficult for a layman to implement so that "OptimiX" has summarized it in some easy-to-understand rules.

Three Rules

"OptimiX" can be summarized in three rules shortly and concisely: - Plant-based foods and beverages: plentiful - Animal foods: moderately - High-fat foods: thrifty with the help of these three rules, parents and adolescents can also eat a full diet.

From these recommendations, one could conclude that nothing is changing much for children with diabetes. But: For those affected, it is different. Suddenly everyone asks: "How much do you want to eat?", "Does the fish contain carbohydrates?" Times become important, and great knowledge of the topic of food is necessary. This is the crucial difference between children with diabetes and children who do not have

diabetes. Diabetics can't just eat as others can. For example, you need to know. B how many carbohydrates a meal has and how the carbohydrates affect blood sugar. They have to think about their food before they bite into a piece of cake or a pizza. Detailed diet plans with an indication of calorie intake, nutrient distribution, or carbohydrate amount are therefore no longer required for normal-weight diabetics. Children, adolescents, and their parents should maintain their previous eating habits or switch to a full-fledged diet. Diabetes therapy should adapt to the everyday life of the children and not the other way around.

And what do children with diabetes eat?

Simply put nothing more than other children who eat a healthy diet! BE and KE – Treasures Carbohydrates play a decisive role in the diet.

Type 1 diabetics must assess the carbohydrates of food to determine the required amount of insulin. The carbohydrate content of a food is subject to a natural fluctuation so that an exact calculation of carbohydrates (KH) is superfluous. In addition, a good blood sugar adjustment can also be achieved with an estimator such as the BE (bread unit) or KE (carbohydrate unit), which corresponds to 10 to 12 grams of carbohydrates. For this reason, an estimate of carbohydrates in the form of BE or KE is sufficient. They are treasures. However, the term estimator does not (only) refer to the fluctuation range of carbohydrates in the food, but also the handling of this unit. Diabetics should be able to estimate their carbohydrate amount. In practice, this means that portions of food should not be weighed, but estimated. Certainly, initially, it is necessary to weigh pasta, potatoes, or strawberries. Only in this way can children and parents develop a feeling for quantities and safely estimate the BE/KE quantity, e.B one portion of potatoes. But the scales must not become a constant companion in everyday life.

Sense and nonsense of diabetic products In modern diabetes therapy, with very few exceptions, there is no justification for the use of diabetic or diet products.

This is pointed out by the Diabetes and Nutrition Group (EASD, 1995) and the German Diabetes Society, among others. Many diabetic foods contain large amounts of fat and energy. They are often more expensive than regular products. In the case of children and adolescents, it should also be noted that when using diabetic products, they may find themselves in a special role vis-à-vis their friends or classmates. A visit to an ice cream parlor or a children's birthday party with cakes and sweets can then quickly lead to an exclusionary situation. Furthermore, compliance with the implementation of the dietary recommendation "optimized mixed food" is not promoted, but rather hindered. A few diabetic foods such as calorie-free sweeteners, light drinks, or sugar-free candies can be useful. So children and adolescents with diabetes can eat a "normal" scoop of ice cream or a chocolate bar sweetened with sucrose.

Training

For children and adolescents with diabetes, training is a central measure of diabetes therapy.

It enables the optimization of blood glucose levels and improves the quality of life. In principle, a distinction must be made in training measures between initial training in the event of the manifestation of diabetes and follow-up training. In the initial training, children and their parents learn the basic skills to deal with diabetes in everyday life. You will learn, for example. B, which foods contain carbohydrates, how meals are estimated, or how carbohydrates affect blood sugar.

Follow-up training courses are used for deepening and repetition and are usually carried out as group training in contrast to the initial training.

Who is being trained?

In this question, it is important to consider how old the child is and who looks after it in everyday life. In small children, the parents (possibly relatives, childminder) play the central role, as they carry out the therapy. From school age onwards, children are increasingly involved in the treatment, so that the children must also be trained. For follow-up training, this means different forms of training, e.B. for primary school children (6 to 10 years), children aged 11 to 13 years, adolescents aged 14 to 16 years, and adolescents aged 17 to 19 years. These transitions in such a division are fluid, and individual stages of development must be taken into account.

Group training – follow-up training is usually offered in small groups and requires differentiated training concepts for different age groups and abilities of the children.

Outpatient training courses offer a good opportunity to train in everyday life, given the proximity to home and motivation of the families. Stationary training offers can also be taken advantage of by families who have a longer journey. They can be an opportunity for less motivated families. The training courses require age-appropriate content education, which is only made possible by a treatment team with both pediatric and dialectological experience.

What is being trained?

Primary school children learn what foods are available, which of them contain carbohydrates and what foods they can eat without calculation. Here, the focus of the training is on imparting practical knowledge. It is also important for children to know that they are not alone in their diabetes.

Schoolchildren deepen their knowledge of what foods contain BEs/KEs. They estimate the corresponding quantities. They are taught knowledge about healthy nutrition and they get to know the different types of carbohydrates and their effect on blood sugar.

For young people, the focus of the training is on greater independence and personal responsibility for their diabetes. This is about topics such as fast food, sweets, alcohol, treatment of hypoglycemia, school trips. But also about background knowledge, e.B. "Why does glucose cause the blood sugar to rise quickly?", "What happens if you eat something?" or "What role do proteins and fats play?".

What is the training done with?

The training material used must be adapted to the age and stage of development of the children. Various training programs can also be used in group training. Appreciating BE and KE can be practiced in conjunction with meals together or with the help of food photos, packaging, or dummies. Children can try carbohydrates in powder form and recognize the differences. Cooking together conveys simply that healthy food can also taste delicious. Collages can be created, recipes calculated or sweets can be examined for their amount of sugar. Helpful are worksheets that accompany the lessons and are also suitable for looking up at home.

Last but not least, children and adolescents with diabetes can eat anything. For them, the same recommendations for a full-fledged diet apply to metabolically healthy children. The prerequisites for this are intensified insulin therapy and a great deal of knowledge about the topic of "eating and drinking". This knowledge must be imparted to families by an experienced treatment team, taking into account the abilities of each family member.

Intensive therapy: imitate nature!

Intensified insulin therapy and insulin pump therapy are now the standard therapy for type 1 diabetics – and also the desirable therapy for active and young type 2 diabetics. Nevertheless, some diabetics ask themselves again and again: "Can't I stay with two syringes a day?" Sure, dangers of in-depth remedy are the multiple injections a day, the mathematics, the frequent blood glucose tests. But there are also weighty advantages: More on this in the following article.

Intensified insulin therapy or ICT has many names: it is also called "basic bolus therapy", by some "functional insulin therapy".

It includes repeated daily insulin injections, in addition, basal and meal-related insulin are strictly separated. The aim of intensified insulin therapy is and was to imitate the function of a healthy pancreas and the beta cells in it as well as possible.

ICT mimics the pancreas Some therefore occasionally speak of "insulin substitution close to the norm".

The pancreas of non-diabetic releases a few units of insulin around the clock every few minutes to meet the body's basic needs for insulin (muscles, adipose tissue, liver, etc.). With meals, additional required amounts of insulin are released, corresponding to the number of carbohydrates consumed as "meal insulin". In healthy people, blood sugar is always kept in the normal range. Type 1 diabetics no longer have their insulin and have to supply this insulin from the outside via a needle, using a pen, a syringe, or even a pump.

The results of the American DCCT study ("Diabetes Control and Complications Trial") published in Boston in 1993 clearly show that the transition from conventional to intensified insulin therapy can dramatically reduce diabetic secondary diseases: diseases of the small vessels, nerves, eyes, and kidneys.

The therapy brings a good quality of life The data were the basis for the fact that intensified insulin therapy must now be regarded as the best possible form of treatment for type 1 diabetics - and also for many type 2 diabetics.

In the DCCT, the quality of life was only marginally examined, but in Germany, it is considered one of the main reasons for the high acceptance of intensified insulin therapy. The big advantage is that meals can be postponed and fixed BE quantities no longer have to be adhered to. Therefore, it is necessary to know the respective insulin requirements for breakfast, lunch, and dinner as well as possibly snacks.

The insulin requirement in type 1 diabetics How do you calculate the insulin requirement as a type 1 diabetic under intensified insulin therapy?

Here are some rules of thumb: - About 0.5 - 1 IU ("International Units") per kg of body weight per day = total daily insulin requirement;

of which about 50 percent normal insulin and 50 percent basal insulin;

distribution of normal insulin to the 3 main meals normally in the ratio of 40:30:30;

The distribution of basal insulin (NPH insulin) usually 50 percent in the morning or at noon and 50 percent at night (bed-time insulin).

When using insulin glargine as basal insulin, a single dose is usually sufficient, no matter what time of day: the need for basal insulin in 24 hours = about half of the total daily amount of insulin: z.B. Total daily dose of insulin: 40 IU, basal insulin requirement: about 20 IU. Due to the different insulin sensitivity in the morning, noon and evening, we need more insulin for breakfast for 1 BE than at noon and in the evening. Therefore, there are different BE factors for breakfast, lunch, and dinner, but also for snacks: The insulin requirement with meals (= prandial insulin requirement / BE factor): in the morning about 1.0 - 3.0 IE / BE, at noon about 0.5 - 1.5 IE / BE, in the evening about 1.0 - 2.0 IE / BE.

The correction factors an IE normal insulin lowers blood sugar depending on individual insulin sensitivity and time of day by about 20 mg/dl to 60 mg/dl (1.1 - 3.2 mmol/l).

A BE of carbohydrates usually raises blood sugar levels by about 20 - 60 mg/dl (1.1 - 3.2 mmol/l).

If you have tested this based on repeated blood glucose measurements before and two to three hours after meals or after correction, nothing stands in the way of a flexible life: with a better quality of life, a reduced risk of hypoglycemia, and a good perspective for the future.

Insulins: large selection for intensified insulin therapy, as for conventional insulin therapy, there are numerous highly purified human insulins;

the list is supplemented by the short-term analog insulin Lispro and insulin Aspart as well as the new long-term analog insulin glargine, which attempts to cover the basal rate by a single subcutaneous injection.

Anyone who uses intensified insulin therapy and uses delay insulin (NPH insulin) with a duration of action of about 8 to 12 hours must usually inject it in the morning and before bedtime (as "bedtime"

insulin). However, in many type 1 diabetics, basal insulin injections are also required at noon, occasionally even in the early evening hours, to bridge the time until the bedtime injection. It is these frequent injections that have led to the desire of many patients to finally develop long-term insulin that only needs to be injected once.

Healthy diet & reasonable weight - With insulin therapy: break weight gain!

Many people with diabetes who start with intensified conventional insulin therapy ("ICT") are gaining significant weight; also because you can now eat what you want - sugarier foods are on the table and fast food. In addition, many still have meat, sausages, and cheeses as well as alcohol, because they can be consumed insulin-independent, are popular with many. And the older you get, the less you move – but the eating habits remain the same; the weight increases insidiously, and since the insulin acts worse with every pound on the ribs, the amounts of insulin become larger and larger.

The advantages and health benefits of intensified insulin therapy are undisputed, as in the long term it significantly reduces the rate of diseases of the small vessels, the rate of secondary diseases of the eyes and kidneys. But many people who use this therapy complain about the load with the kilos: "I have gained significantly!

Losing weight successfully: the first steps Check your eating habits.

Fat is a calorie bomb (1 gram provides 9 calories). If you eat more low-fat, you can save a lot of fat calories. The amount of bread topping or the size of the meat portion also plays a "greasy" role: Many people think "It's low in fat – you can take more", but protein also provides calories! And: Do not drink as much alcohol, because it provides almost as many calories as fat! Overweight diabetics should hardly or if possible not eat sugary foods, because they are bad if you want to reduce your weight; of course, chocolate is delicious, you don't have to treat yourself to a whole bar – some ribs do it too. Increase the daily amounts of vegetables and salad, they make you full and provide few calories.

Helps!

Anyone who has become a bit rusty over the years due to lack of exercise or has never been particularly athletic should start with light activities: Untrained people with diabetes can hypoglycemia faster and should not underestimate the effect of walks if they have otherwise moved little. Planning is the be-all and end-all to save insulin and not to eat "after" the movement.

Sometimes you have miscalculated and not reduced enough insulin, so that quickly effective carbohydrates are required. Physical activity accelerates the transport of glucose to the muscle cell and leads to a reduction in insulin requirements. However, the type, duration, and time of movement are always very decisive: If you are unsure about insulin adaptation, you should work it out together with your doctor/diabetes consultant.

Running, cycling, hiking: all good for you!

You will learn every day through your own experience and blood glucose measurements; in addition, each person reacts differently. Many endurance sports such as walking, hiking, walking, running, cycling or swimming improve blood circulation - the insulin works better, can be reduced, and they very effectively support weight loss; a special treat is provided by the sports mentioned: You do almost all of them in the fresh air, they are cost-effective and time-independent. Even without insulin reduction, physical activities can support weight loss, possibly low blood sugar levels can be compensated by glucose or fruit. People who exercise persistently two to three times a week (30 to 60 minutes) have significantly fewer weight problems.

Additional energy consumption through 30 minutes of Movement

sport	Energy consumption in kcal
Walking (4 km/h)	75 to 95
Walking (8 km/h)	140 to 175
Jogging/running (12 km/h)	185 to 230
Light gymnastics	85 to 105
Backstroke (1.2 km/h)	165 to 210
Cycling (21 km/h)	190 to 245

Too much insulin? Check more often!

You should regularly check whether your basal insulin dose and your dose for eating are still correctly selected. Many people with diabetes inject 40 to 50 percent of the daily insulin requirement as delayed insulin: If you overdose with basal insulin, you will be forced to eat more carbohydrates during the day. Are you one of those people with diabetes who eat as little BE/KE as possible, but more meat, sausage, or cheese? Then you need over 50 percent basal insulin. Unfortunately, it is the BE/KE savers who have the most weight problems, as they satisfy their hunger with meat and sausage. In some diabetics, the basal insulin requirement is very different during the day and at night; there are different tests, depending on the type of insulin, to determine the right need. Most miscalculations happen when eating. Even experienced diabetics underestimate or overestimate the carbohydrate content of a meal and eat possibly too much injected insulin afterward. Often the BE/KE factors are not right, which can also change over the years.

Is fasting a Solution?

In the case of weight loss, the need for insulin changes considerably and it must be adjusted; fasting is also possible. If you want to fast for a day, then inject only the delayed insulin and a small amount (5 percent of the daily insulin) of short-acting insulin in the morning. After about ten to twelve hours, the blood sugar can drop a bit, and you should eat some glucose (2 to 3 BE / KE) throughout the day to stabilize. By fasting, the liver releases less glucose. If you want to fast for more days, you should lower the delayed insulin in 10 percent increments. Close-meshed blood glucose self-checks are extremely important here. However, fasting - in the sense of the inventor - is not a suitable method to reduce weight. Eating, drinking, and exercise habits must be changed in small steps to successfully reduce weight permanently.

The conclusion You can break the continuous weight gain with many years of ICT.

I would like to encourage you because in our clinic I experience again and again how by changing the insulin therapy, the diet and with a little more exercise, the pounds melt and the blood sugar values improve.

All about insulin

When does insulin therapy make sense for people with type 2 diabetes? And what requirements must be met? More about this in the following article.

Before starting insulin therapy, structured diabetes training should take place: In terms of content, those affected should learn all the basics necessary for insulin therapy; of course, blood glucose self-measurements should then also be learned and carried out regularly. If you regularly log your blood glucose levels, this will give your doctor a good overview of the current blood glucose setting and facilitate the necessary dose adjustments. The self-injection of insulin and the handling of insulin injection aids (pens) should be practiced and controlled. If the person concerned is not able to inject insulin himself, either relative must be trained or a nursing service must be called in. The insulin type insulin is a protein hormone composed of 51 amino acids and formed in the B cells of the pancreas.

It primarily regulates sugar metabolism, but also fat and protein metabolism. Depending on the level of blood sugar, its release is stimulated or slowed down as required.

The first artificially produced insulins in the 20s of the last century were obtained from animal-bellies salivary glands of pigs or cattle. The difference to human insulin (human insulin) is only one in pigs and three amino acids in cattle. This explains the same metabolic effect on the cells, but because of the different protein structure in some patients also a certain number of intolerance reactions against this animal insulin. Today, only human insulins or insulin analogs are used for insulin control (i.e. genetically modified insulins).

Short-acting human insulins

The short-acting human insulins (normal insulin, old insulin) have an effective duration of three to five hours: They are therefore suitable as meal insulins.

After injection into the subcutaneous fatty tissue, its effect begins after about 15 to 30 minutes, which is why a spray-eating distance should be maintained from 0 to 30 minutes depending on the level of blood sugar before the meal. The main effect takes place after the 2nd to 3rd hour. Fast- and short-acting insulin analogs an insulin analog is a human insulin molecule that has different properties than the starting product of human insulin due to genetic modification of the amino acid sequence or its protein structure; in the case of the fast- and short-acting insulin analogs, the self-binding of the individual analog molecules is lower by a change in the amino acid sequence; as a result, the molecules enter the blood circulation faster? Consequence: The effect starts faster after the injection. The total duration of action is shorter with two to three hours compared to conventional human insulin, but still longer than the effect of the body's insulin (see the table? Duration of action and kinetics of action of insulins?).

The maximum action is reached after just one hour. Due to these properties, the short-acting insulin analogs usually do not require an injection-eating distance. At low baseline values before the meal, even to avoid hypoglycemia, it is necessary to inject only after eating. At higher initial values before the meal, however, a spray-eating interval of 10 to 30 minutes is also appropriate here. Short-acting insulin analogs should not be reared together with delayed insulins, both insulins should be injected separately.

The short-acting insulins are due to their short, limited duration of action only suitable for the metabolism of meals. Delay and baseline lines.

For the basic insulin requirement required between meals and during the night, lower insulin concentrations are required compared to the meal requirement, which is covered by basal or delay insulins.

If human insulin is coupled to certain substances, e.B. protamine, an insulin-protamine complex with an extended duration of action is formed. These NPH insulins (neutral protamine Hagedorn insulin) act for about 8 to 12 hours depending on the amount injected but still have a pronounced maximum effect after 4 to 7 hours. This property of baseline saline can cause hypoglycemia, especially at night, but also during the day.

Lente insulins

In the insulin group of Lente insulins, the effect of insulin is prolonged by a higher zinc concentration. In Germany, insulin semblance (pig insulin) is occasionally used even if the NPH insulin does not work long enough over the night in the early morning hours. The delays described above are turbid suspensions and must be carefully mixed before use. This is especially true when, as is usually the case, insulin pens are used for injection.

Long-acting insulin

Analogs Insulin glargine is a genetically modified human insulin whose change in the amino acid structure has led to the extension of the duration of action to approx. 24 hours. It is clear insulin with acidic pH and usually only needs to be injected once a day due to its long duration of action. Insulin glargine can not be mixed with other insulins. It has no pronounced maximum effect and is therefore particularly suitable as basic insulin? combined with normal insulin or short-acting insulin analogs, but also as a combination partner in the treatment with tablets.

Genetic engineering: side effects?

In recent years, a controversial discussion has been held in Germany about the side effects or dangers of genetically engineered insulins. The short-acting insulin analogs have now been in use worldwide for about five years, without any serious side effects being observed. It can therefore be assumed that their application satisfies the high-security requirements of the authorities.

In the case of long-acting insulin analogs (insulin glargine), such a long period of use is not yet overlooked. We refer to the detailed discussion regarding possible dangers in the issue 3/2001. Mixed insulins and combination analogs Mixed insulins are finished insulin mixtures that are composed of two components:

a) the fast-acting portion - normal insulin or a - short-acting insulin analog
b) the delay component with basal or NPH insulin.

With two doses a day, the fast-acting portion of the morning dose should cover breakfast, the delay portion the morning, lunch, and afternoon. The evening dose is intended for metabolization of dinner and to cover the nocturnal base insulin requirement. Most often, the mixture is used 25 percent (30 percent) of normal insulin or short-acting insulin analog and 75 percent (70 percent) of basal insulin. For patients with a large breakfast or high insulin requirement in the morning, the mixture is available with 50 percent normal insulin or short-acting insulin analog and 50 percent delayed insulin. Mixed insulins are mainly used in conventional insulin therapy.

Contraindications to insulin are not known; the main side effect of insulin administration is hypoglycemia (hypoglycemia) - hypoglycemia occurs with overdoses of single insulin or with overlapping of effects and summation of two different insulins: Z.B. the morning normal insulin effect overlaps with the effect of the morning basal insulin and then leads to hypoglycemia around 11 o'clock. Another danger of insulin treatment is weight gain in type 2 diabetics. Especially if insulin is used in too high a dosage, is the danger of? Insulin fattening? Given that, the patient gains weight. Other causes of hypoglycemia may be increased physical or sporting activity or meals misjudged or omitted about their carbohydrate content. Change the injection points in the event of non-replacement of the injection sites, i.e. if repeatedly injected into the same site, it can lead to loss of fatty tissue (Lipoatrophy) or adipose tissue/connective tissue formation (Lipoatrophy).

Insulin release from such places is disturbed. The insulin effect is then no longer calculable. For this reason, the injection points should be changed daily. Real allergies to insulin are rare.

Diabetes and smoking: ominous!

People are at risk because they have diabetes alone - about circulatory disorders of the coronary vessels, the brain-supplying arteries, but also the leg arteries. Circulatory disorders are also a special danger for very strongly perfused organs such as the kidney and very "oxygen-sensitive" regions such as the retina of the eyes. Many risk factors such as high blood pressure, lipid metabolism disorders, and also obesity worsen blood circulation – and a special, avoidable risk factor is smoking!

No other "stimulant" has a comparably strong influence on the overall mortality of people in Germany, which is why preventive measures in particular – i.e. not to start smoking in the first place – should have a high priority. Most smokers start smoking in adolescence or early adulthood, with habituation and dependence over time leading to the continuation of tobacco consumption. Most smokers themselves know about the health hazard, but many sometimes consciously take the risk: they often rate the positive consequences of smoking higher than the negative ones or feel dependent on nicotine.

Immediately...

About half of all young smokers cite immediate satisfaction from smoking as a motive – "because I like to smoke", "because I like it", "because it calms me down"; these attitudes are also reflected in advertising.

About 25 to 50 percent of young smokers also cite social reasons ("smoking infects"). For many young people, social norms, the behavior

of role models, and also the pressure in the reference group of young people (peer group) also play an important role in the onset of smoking. However, the group effect can also promote non-smoking. With regular smoking, in many cases, a dependency eventually occurs in the habituation, which often makes it difficult to quit smoking.

... And makes you sick!

In addition to the aforementioned circulatory disorders, which are mainly caused by nicotine, smoking is blamed for several other diseases: Cancer in the form of lung cancer and diseases of the respiratory organs, especially in the form of chronic bronchitis. But also the appearance of stomach ulcers, the significantly reduced birth weight of children in smokers, and the sudden infant death are mentioned in connection with smoking. In combination with alcohol, there is an increased risk of oral cavity cancer. And smokers who take the "birth control pill" at the same time have a significantly increased risk of thrombosis. In addition, there are very special risks for diabetics (see info box).

The total mortality rate, which is attributed to smoking for individual diseases, is in some cases up to 90 percent. The risk of lung cancer is more than 20 times higher in male smokers, the risk of throat cancer more than 10 times higher than in non-smokers. More than 80 to 90 percent of the risk of lung cancer and laryngeal cancer is attributed to smoking. It is estimated that in Germany at present between 90 000 and 140 000 people a year die as a result of tobacco consumption. Ultimately, it does not matter whether you smoke cigarettes on the lungs or just "puff" cigarillos or cigars or pipes: In any case, the nicotine harmful to the vessels is absorbed via the oral mucosa.

Even passive smoking: dangerous!

We now know that passive smoking, in other words, involuntary inhalation of tobacco smoke, also has a very negative impact on human health. It is known that, especially in old age, children up to 5 years of age have more acute and chronic diseases of the respiratory organs if they are regularly exposed to tobacco smoke in the family by parents or other relatives. It is also known in adults that passive smoking causes and sustains respiratory diseases. The risk of coronary heart disease and lung cancer also appears to have increased.

But how to stop?

Many smokers need professional support to quit smoking in the short or long term. The chances of success are generally higher if it is a lighter form of smoking than a pronounced dependence. And the prospects are good if no previous attempts at weaning have been made and the motivation is particularly high. Maximum professional therapists work behaviorally due to the fact the natural drug treatment techniques cannot damage via sure behaviors that allows you to cease smoking immediately.

Chewing gum and patches help temporarily Today, nicotine replacement preparations, which are available, for example, like nicotine gum, nicotine patches, or nicotine spray, can temporarily support; as a rule, the concept is tailored in such a way that the amount of nicotine in the patch or chewing gum is reduced weekly to gradually wean. Both the patch and the chewing gum are available without a prescription in the pharmacy. However, all these measures must necessarily be carried out with the attending physician and not in the form of self-therapy. As previously described, nicotine leads to vasoconstriction, so that the combination of chewing gum and plaster can already have a vasoconstrictive effect and thus lead to damage - their use is therefore not completely unproblematic. Therefore, all nicotine replacement preparations are limited in their period of application to about 6 months. Of course, it is best if you can cope without nicotine substitutes - and without withdrawal symptoms such as irritability, palpitations, fatigue, and impaired concentration.

Behavioral therapy: Avoid cigarette smoke!

Behavioral therapeutic approaches take into account, for example, that you avoid societies in which people smoke regularly - for example, pub visits; and that you occasionally reward yourself for your nicotine abstinence, but not with a cigarette; and that they especially take the opportunity to start again with endurance sports and activity in the great outdoors - think e.B. of cycling, gardening. You will ultimately be rewarded with the fact that first of all your clothes and the apartment no longer smell of nicotine, the sense of taste and smell is sharpened again and you notice again how nice it is to breathe in the fresh air outdoors...

It's schizophrenic...

All this with the certainty that after about 10 to 15 years, even in previous smokers, the risk of lung cancer and heart attack, but also circulatory disorders, will approach that of a non-smoker again. Smoking cessation training, as we also offer in our clinic, should ultimately help to persuade every diabetic who still smokes to stop this habit or dependence, which is harmful to him, as soon as possible.

Often enough I have to stress to patients that we are not against smokers, but against smoking: because it seems schizophrenic that we do everything possible to better permeate the blood vessels, especially in diabetics - and on the other hand, patients often deliberately narrow their vessels several times a day, some even 1/2 hour. Non-smoking should be one of his top goals for the future for every diabetic!

Type 2 diabetes – or rather "insulin resistance disease"

The finding that diabetes mellitus type 2 is also a vascular disease seems to be contrary to the previously usual definition of this clinical picture. Diabetes is considered a metabolic disease in which a more or less pronounced deficiency of endogenous insulin mainly affects the metabolism of carbohydrates and lipids.

Damage to the vascular system is possible as micro- and macroangiopathies. Microangiopathy occurs on the smallest vessels. Their appearance is diabetic retinopathy, nephropathy, and neuropathy. Macroangiopathy can manifest itself on the coronary vessels and lead to a heart attack. It can affect the cerebral vessels and cause an apoplectic insult, and it can cause a peripheral arterial occlusion disease in the event of an infestation of the limb arteries.

Vascular lesions not a complication, but a symptom in publications on diabetic vascular lesions, the term "vascular complications" can still be found today.

This gives the impression that these are the consequences of a particularly unfavorable, complicated process.

However, type 2 diabetes is fatefully accompanied by such vascular wall changes. Diabetic Angiopathy is therefore not a complication, but a disease-defining and prognosis-determining symptom.

Coronary heart disease is twice as common in diabetics as in non-diabetics. The risk of infarction in diabetics is much greater for both the first infarction and a pure infarction than for non-diabetic patients. Diabetics also have a lower chance of survival after a heart attack than non-diabetics.

The cardiovascular mortality risk of diabetics is 2 to 6 times higher than in non-diabetics. Overall, more than 80% of all diabetics die as a result of progressive atherosclerosis.

The dominance of cardiovascular events in the course of type 2 diabetes has led to a new definition of this clinical picture. Today, diabetes is considered a high-risk cardiovascular disease in which blood sugar is also elevated.

Thus, the diabetic vascular lesions receive at least the same importance as the carbohydrate metabolism disorder. For a long time, the interaction of insulin and blood sugar alone was the focus of diagnostic and therapeutic interest.

Pathogenesis of type 2 diabetes The close relationships between lifestyle habits, genetic stress as well as resulting metabolic behavior and vascular changes are recorded in a scheme of multifactorial pathogenesis of type 2 diabetes.

According to recent findings, insulin resistance is at the heart of the pathogenetic mechanisms that eventually lead to the manifestation of type 2 diabetes.

The course of the disease in the diabetic course of the disease, a distinction is made between prediabetes, in which a laboratory-chemically detectable "disturbed glucose tolerance" occurs only in its final stage, and the actual manifest diabetes.

At the beginning of the prediabetic disease, the phase is insulin resistance. Almost simultaneously, endothelial dysfunction, hyperlipoproteinemia, and hypertensive circulatory dysregulation develop. The consequence of this risk constellation is atherosclerotic vascular wall changes, even before the detection of a "disturbed glucose tolerance".

It should be borne in mind, if the diabetic course of the disease in its early stages goes back to the manifest insulin resistance, whether the combined occurrence of vascular lesions and metabolic disorders should not be called an "insulin resistance disease" from the outset. The fact that the vascular lesions in type 2 diabetes are not only of theoretical and scientific importance is proven by the results of the recently published HYDRA study.

On a cut-off date in 2001, all patients who visited the 1912 practices involved in this study were examined for obesity, hypertension, and diabetes. The result of the study was a high incidence of hypertension and a conspicuous coincidence of hypertension and diabetes mellitus. For example, in a total of 45,000 patients, hypertension was detected in every second patient, diabetes mellitus in every fifth patient, and a joint occurrence of hypertension and diabetes in every tenth case of treatment.

The causes of vascular lesions in type 2 diabetes are complex. According to recent studies, it is especially the postprandial increase in blood sugar that increases the risk of vascular lesions typical of diabetes. In addition, there are disorders of endothelial function, the diabetic pathological lipid profile as well as lipo- and glucotoxicity.

The STOP-NIDDM study has shown that the attenuation or even prevention of postprandial excessive blood sugar increase by long-term administration of 3 x 100 mg acarbose reduces the occurrence of cardiovascular events by 49% compared to a placebo collective. The conversion of impaired glucose tolerance into manifest type 2 diabetes was reduced by 36%, and the incidence of heart attacks in the collective treated with acarbose was even 91% lower than in the placebo group.

In addition to the reduction of postprandial hyperglycemia, these treatment successes are also due to the influence of post-elementary lipid metabolism and the influence on the formation of free radicals, insulin resistance, sympathicotonia, and endothelial dysfunction. In practice, the long-term use of such a high dose of acarbose is likely to be only partially practicable due to possible gastrointestinal side effects.

Insulin resistance and obesity Insulin resistance is detectable in more than 90% of obese type 2 diabetics.

It can be treated and is reversible. Thus, insulin resistance can be reduced and reduced by a healthier lifestyle, by a long-term change in nutritional behavior with healthy, fat-restricted food and a gradual weight loss favored with it, as well as by a regular, individually adapted, if possible forced exercise and physical activity.

Two prevention studies prove how effective a change in the "lifestyle" alone can be: In the Finnish "Diabetes Prevention Study", two patient groups of a total of 522 patients with impaired glucose tolerance were observed over five years. The Verum group was advised in detail about necessary changes in their way of life and a restriction of fat consumption to 30%, while saturated fats below 10%, as well as a weight loss of more than 5% and regular physical training of 30 minutes daily demanded. The placebo group received only standard counseling. At the end of the study, the cumulative incidence of diabetes in the Verum group was 58% lower than in the comparison collective.

Effectively combating obesity, The American "Diabetes Prevention Program" comes to the same results. 3234 patients with "impaired glucose tolerance" were divided into three groups. In one group, repeated dietary consultation and prescription of an individual diet with limited fat intake took place. Weight loss by more than 7% and a weekly physical workout of 150 minutes were the success criteria. The second group of patients was advised only as standard and additionally received metformin. The third group, in turn, was taught only in a standardized way.

Here, too, the risk of diabetes in the "active-life-style" group was reduced by 58% and in the metformin group by 31% compared to the standard collective.

The change in lifestyle habits, but above all the effective fight against obesity, is, therefore, a recipe for success in reducing insulin resistance with its effects on metabolic behavior and cardiovascular prognosis.

Therapy of type 2 diabetes If insulin resistance continues with its effects on the metabolic process and the vascular system, the exclusive treatment of the KH metabolic disorder or the sole therapy of impaired fat metabolism, endothelial dysfunction and hypertension would only be a symptomatic procedure.

Rather, all these facets of insulin resistance must be treated with equal intensity.

The angiotensinogen formed in the liver is converted by renin into angiotensin I. Under the influence of ACE (angiotensin-converting enzyme), angiotensin II is formed. For the effectiveness of angiotensin II, there are two receptors among several subtypes, the AT-1 receptor, and the AT-2 receptor, to which the angiotensin II can dock. Via the AT-1 receptor, angiotensin II develops its blood pressure-enhancing effectiveness.

The ACE inhibitors cause by influencing the angiotensin-converting enzyme a reduced formation of angiotensin II and thus a weakening of vasoconstriction. At the same time, ACE inhibitors reduce the degradation

of the vasodilation bradykinin. It is noteworthy that ace inhibitors reduce the formation of angiotensin II only by about 20-30%. 70-80% of angiotensin II are formed directly from angiotensinogen by mediating the enzyme chymase.

If the AT-1 receptor is partially blocked by Sarton's, which are also referred to as AT-1 receptor blockers or, more broadly, angiotensin II antagonists, angiotensin II docks to the AT-2 receptor. This leads to the increased formation of bradykinin, a vasodilator. The Sarton thus not only weakens the vasoconstrictive effect of angiotensin II but also indirectly promotes vasodilation by bradykinin.

The different targets of Sarton and ACE inhibitors on the RAS system make a combined application of both active ingredients to reduce blood pressure seem particularly promising. The results of the recently completed VALIANT study will provide information on this.

Conclusion

The new findings on the active metabolic function of the endothelium as well as on the early inflammatory processes in the development of atherosclerosis, on disorders of fat metabolism, on the causes of hypertension, and finally on the homeostasis of fibrinolysis and ant fibrinolytic have led to a different evaluation of the vascular manifestations in type 2 diabetes.

Type 2 diabetes is a mosaic of pathological changes that no longer warrants the previous focus on blood glucose behavior as a standard of therapy and prognosis. The term "diabetes" has long since lost its literal meaning. Rather, it is the clinical effects of insulin resistance, the "metabolic syndrome", that shape the clinical picture of type 2 diabetes.

This raises the question of whether the diabetic KH metabolic disorder is not only one of several facets of the metabolic syndrome. Then the accompanying hypolipoproteinemia would not be a precursor of the diabetic disease, but an (early) symptom of an "insulin resistance disease". Also, the premature and accelerated occurring atherosclerotic vascular lesions would no longer be diabetes-specific fateful. Rather, the added KH metabolic disorder would only be a catalyst for atherosclerosis progression in an "insulin resistance disease".

With the introduction of the term "insulin resistance disease", the previous division into diabetes mellitus type 1 and 2 would become obsolete. It has long been known that these two diseases are so different that they only have a name in common. Likewise, the clinically and laboratory chemically inhomogeneous concept of disease of "prediabetes" would be superfluous. Finally, the term "insulin resistance disease" would more convincingly justify the global treatment concept to be practiced in the future.

Regardless of such speculation, it must already be a therapeutic consequence to treat type 2 diabetes not only in a blood sugar-oriented manner. Rather, disorders of lipid metabolism, hypertensive circulatory dysregulation, and endothelial dysfunction must be treated equally and equitably in favor of atherosclerosis prophylaxis.

Type 2 diabetes and hypertension: from expert opinion to evidence

In the past ten years, it has become clear worldwide that patients with type 2 diabetes are extremely likely to have hypertension. Contrary to a long-popular idea, it is not to be seen and treated as a late consequence of nephropathy, but as a rule as an early partial symptom of insulin resistance syndrome. Evidence-based medicine has now also produced useful study data for diabetes patients with hypertension. Until a few years ago, the recommendations of the professional societies for the treatment of hypertension in type 2 diabetes were based on an analogy, in the absence of studies, in that data collected from non-diabetics or undiagnosed diabetics were transferred to diabetes patients. This was because in the earlier hypertension intervention studies, the characteristic diabetes was generally defined as an exclusion criterion and existing data on diabetic subgroups were difficult to interpret for methodological reasons. It was only with the publication of the UKPD study and the HOT and HOPE data that due attention was paid to the hypertensive patients with the acknowledged highest cardiovascular risk – namely those with type 2 diabetes.

Paradigm shift, change in values, and a drop in limit values According to the current criteria of the Joint National Committee on Detection, Evaluation, and Treatment of High Blood Pressure (JNC-VI), blood pressure above 140/90 mmHg is considered elevated.

Approximately 15-25% of the European population exceeds this limit, but 80% of patients with type 2 diabetes. Especially in this population group, however, the following is no longer the sole measure of things for the individual therapy decision. According to the JNC-VI guidelines, two questions, in particular, are of central importance: Is there hypertensive end-organ damage or atherosclerosis?

Are there other cardiovascular risk factors?

Patients with type 2 diabetes usually have a whole bundle of other risk factors in addition to the increased blood pressure, so that the active search is always worthwhile.

Figure 1 shows both the relevant end-organ damage and the risk factors. It is noticeable that diabetes patients are obligately in the group with the highest risk to be treated with medication.

The individual partial symptoms of insulin resistance syndrome are usually networked and interdependent in a complex way and are present long before the respective clinical diagnosis of hypertension or type 2 diabetes. Persons with insulin resistance syndrome already have an extraordinarily high risk of atherosclerosis based on this combination of risk factors already in the prediabetic stage, without this having been sufficiently taken into account in therapeutic strategies so far. The concept of treating essential hypertension as part of a bundle of risk factors with possibly common etiology (i.e. insulin resistance syndrome) has important implications for cardiovascular primary and secondary prevention and risk factor management. Among the non-pharmacological measures, a reasonable lifestyle, a reduction in saline and calorie consumption, alcohol and nicotine consumption, an existing overweight and increased physical exercise are the central steps to improve the insulin effect and reduce blood pressure. In drug hypertension therapy, substances that aggravate pre-existing insulin resistance, do not improve the cardiovascular risk profile, and have no evidence for organ protective effects should no longer be administered uncritically. According to prospective study results such as HOPE, the improved insulin effect under ACE inhibitors also appears to be reflected in a more favorable event-free probability of survival compared to other substances and a lower prevalence of diabetes.

Clear data situation versus unclear interpretation The much-cited United Kingdom Prospective Diabetes Study (UKPDS) with its subsequently launched subproject Hypertension in Diabetes Study (HDS) seems to have shown on the superficial view that a tight blood pressure adjustment benefits type 2 diabetes patients and that ACE inhibitors and beta-blockers are equivalent when it comes to preventing complications. The Hypertension in Diabetes Study compared a "taut" and a "less taut" blood pressure setting in terms of clinical endpoints in 1148 patients with type 2 diabetes and hypertension between 1987 and 1996. In the taut group, the beta-blockers atenolol (n = 358) and the ACE inhibitor captopril (n = were used as the first substances. The examined patients were on average 56 years old, were treated with an average initial blood pressure of 160/94 mmHg according to today's ideas in hypertension stage 2, and thus initially inadequately. Diabetes, on the other hand, was well adjusted at an HbA1c of 6.9 and 7.0, respectively, while the mean weight was on the verge of obesity.

For numerous methodological reasons, considerable doubts are justified that USPDS/HDS proves the widespread conclusions mentioned and is suitable as a guideline for medical action in this country.

For example, about 13 and 16% of the participants were people of color, whose metabolic and blood pressure situation is known not to be comparable to that of white Europeans. Only in 78% (captopril) and 65% (atenolol) of the observed patient-years were the corresponding drugs taken. Finally, most of the participants were additionally treated with furosemide, nifedipine, methyldopa, or prazosin.

The surrogate parameters showed that the metabolic adjustment with the ß-blocker was only worse in the first 4 years (HbA1c 7.5 vs. 7.0), which after 8.4 years due to increased antidiabetic treatment (66 vs. 53%) was compensable.

The weight gain was permanently stronger under atenolol (3.4 vs.

1.6 kg). All this did not affect the hard endpoints: An Equieffective reduction in blood pressure was opposed by an equal risk reduction of micro-and microvascular endpoints.

Absurd therapy goal, Unfortunately, most of the numerous study interpreters do not bother to track down the facts behind the terms.

For example, "less tight control" initially meant a therapy goal of <200/105 mmHg, which was mitigated in 1989 into the still absurd therapy goal of <180/105. Under "taut" we have to imagine a therapy goal of <150/85 mmHg, which is also no longer up-to-date given the current ideas on target blood pressure (125-135/75-85 mmHg).

The pressures achieved after 9 years were 144/83 mm/Hg with captopril and 143/81 mm/Hg with atenolol as initial therapy.

Conclusion

The USPD/HDS data were collected at a blood pressure level that is much too high from today's point of view.

The nevertheless convincing results seem to speak for the priority of the general reduction of blood pressure over the individual differential therapeutic consideration.

The apparent equivalence of beta-blockers and ACE inhibitors about clinical endpoints cannot be considered proven due to methodological deficiencies and has now been refuted by several current studies.

For example, through the data of the CAPPP study (Captopril Prevention Project): In this perspective, open study with blinded endpoint analysis, 5493 patients with essential hypertension in the middle age of 52.5 (25-

years were treated with captopril or beta-blockers (plus possibly hydrochlorothiazide plus possibly diltiazem) over an observation period of 6.1 years. In the CAPPP collective, there was also no difference between ACE inhibitors and beta-blockers about the primary combined endpoint of myocardial infarction and stroke (both fatal and non-fatal).

In contrast, in the subgroup of diabetics (n=574), myocardial infarction incidence, the number of cardiovascular deaths, and the combined primary endpoint with the ACE inhibitor were significantly lower than with the beta-blocker.

In addition, the incidence of diabetes (secondary endpoint) in the subgroup of captopril-treated non-diabetics was significantly lower with 6.1% (336/5493) vs. 6.9% (379/5493) (p=0.04), which corresponds to a number needed to treat (NNT) of 111.

Exciting result

This interesting observation was reproduced and expanded shortly afterward by the HOPE study (Heart Outcomes Prevention Evaluation), which had a high proportion of diabetes patients with almost 40%.

In HOPE, the target blood pressure achieved was 140/77 mmHg. Looking at the subgroup of diabetics, not only did the 1808 patients with Ramipril experience fewer heart attacks (NNT 38), cardiovascular deaths (NNT 34), and strokes (NNT 56), but also all-cause mortality (NNT 30) decreased significantly. The even more exciting result, however, refers to the high-pressure patients who did not (yet) have diabetes at the beginning of the study. That was initially just over 60% in each group.

The absolute risk of manifesting diabetes during the observation period was 3.6% with Ramipril (102/2837), but not 5.4% (156/2883). This results in an NNT of 56 and the conclusion that ACE inhibitors are suitable for the primary prevention of type 2 diabetes.

Most interpreters have not yet recognized this result in its scope, many perceived it as a surprise and few expected it as a "proof of principle".

Thus, we and others have already shown in the 80s of the last century that ACE inhibition improves the surrogate parameters of insulin sensitivity and endothelial function.

Since HOPE, the clinical benefit of ACE inhibition has now been proven in this regard.

Non-drug therapy Table 1 shows the current recommendation of the German High-Pressure League for non-drug therapy of increased blood pressure.

Although it does not say so, it is obvious from the context that each of the measures listed improves insulin sensitivity. The causal form of therapy of all aspects of insulin resistance syndrome is to change the way of life. Calorie and reduced-fat diet and weight loss, if necessary, aerobic physical exercise, if possible, improve glucose utilization. Saline restriction, as well as alcohol restriction, reduces both insulin resistance and blood pressure.

Excessive fat and carbohydrate intake raise sympathicotonia. Therefore, it is understandable that a calorie-reduced diet affects insulin sensitivity, insulin levels, and blood pressure synergistically and favorably. Weight reduction also leads to a simultaneous decrease in plasma insulin, norepinephrine concentrations, increased blood sugar and blood pressure. Physical training causes an acute increase in insulin sensitivity via increased muscular glucose oxidation as well as in the medium and long term via improved CA pillarization and an altered fiber distribution of the skeletal muscles. In addition, the concentration of HDL cholesterol increases and blood pressure decreases, which is particularly evident in insulin-resistant people. The fact that blood pressure is associated with salt sensitivity, especially in obese persons, as well as with adrenal stimulation and insulin resistance, has been known for some time. However, salt sensitivity also seems to be coupled with insulin resistance in normal-weight Normotonicians. Saline restriction thus leads to a decrease in blood pressure and an improvement in glucose tolerance in salt-sensitive persons, regardless of weight. Finally, it is now clearly proven that nicotine causes insulin resistance with all the aforementioned metabolic and cardiovascular consequences, which is reversible within a few weeks.

Drug therapy

If, after assessing the risk factors and organ damage, a drug hypertension treatment is indicated, today in the selection of antihypertensive drugs is also no longer only the hypotensive effect in the foreground.

The additional consideration of the influences on the metabolism, the insulin residence syndrome, and the organ protection gains decisive importance for differential therapeutic considerations.

Beta-blockers and thiazide diuretics have not been able to significantly reduce the coronary risk in primary prevention in the past. This has been explained repeatedly by the negative influence on insulin resistance, but this has not yet been proven. That selective beta-blockers in secondary prophylaxis after infarction, especially in diabetics, have a beneficial effect and are not inferior to ace inhibitors in primary prophylaxis (UKPDS) has been proven.

Frequency-neutral or long-acting calcium channel blockers were considered suitable for patients with hypertension in the context of metabolic syndrome, as they do not worsen insulin sensitivity. Non-retarded nifedipine, on the other hand, should no longer be used in metabolic syndrome as well as in the concomitant heart or kidney failure. In two studies, it was surprisingly shown that long-acting calcium channel blockers were also inferior in comparison with ACE inhibitors in terms of cardiovascular event risk.

For ace inhibitors, favorable metabolic effects in the sense of an insulin sensitivity increase of skeletal muscles could be repeatedly demonstrated in essential hypertensive with and without type 2 diabetes. This is a bradykinin-mediated acute effect, which on the one hand stems from the increase in blood circulation in the muscles, on the other hand directly from an increased translocation of muscular glucose transporters. According to current data, ACE inhibition increases glucose utilization in the muscles and thus the insulin effect by about 10 to 20%. According to a meta-analysis of controlled studies, a mean HbA1c drop of 7% is expected in patients with type 2 diabetes under ACE inhibitor treatment. According to the CAPPP and HOPE data, the diabetes risk of hypertensive patients decreases when treated with an ACE inhibitor.

For the alpha-1 blockers, which are no longer the 1st choice since ALLHAT, favorable effects on blood circulation, insulin sensitivity, and Dyslipoproteinemia could also be shown in clinical and experimental studies. However, prospective, endpoint-oriented data on patients with insulin residence syndrome are missing.

Central Antisympathicotonics does not currently appear in the scheme of the high-pressure league. However, imidazole I1 receptor antagonists could help this class of substances to achieve a renaissance, especially in insulin-resistant hypertensive.

The data for AT1 receptor blockers (ARPS) is promising from the point of view of low side effects, metabolic neutrality, and recently also about organ protection.

Thus, ACE inhibitors, selective b-blockers, and ARPS are currently the first choice for patients with hypertension and insulin resistance syndrome.

Whether they can reduce the coronary risk has yet to be proven in future studies. However, initial prospective study results unanimously indicate a lower risk of events.

Summary

The concept of seeing and treating essential hypertension as part of a bundle of risk factors with a potentially common etiology has important implications for primary cardiovascular prevention and risk factor management.

Regardless of the so far unresolved causality question, the insulin resistance concept provides a viable basis for the treatment of hypertension and the prevention of type 2 diabetes and atherosclerosis. Among the non-pharmacological measures, a reasonable lifestyle, a reduction in the consumption of table salt and calories, alcohol and nicotine consumption, an existing overweight and more physical exercise are the central steps to improve the insulin effect and to reduce blood pressure. In drug blood pressure therapy, substances that only lower blood pressure, but aggravate the pre-existing insulin resistance and risk factor profile and have no organ protective effect, should no longer be administered uncritically.

Hypoglycemia problems in diabetes mellitus – Etiology, diagnostics, and treatment

Hypoglycemia problems are an increasing challenge in the treatment of insulin-dependent diabetes patients. The prevalence in type 1 diabetes patients is about 20-30%. Recent studies have shown that hypoglycemia problems can also be relevant in type 2 diabetes patients. The etiology of hypoglycemia-associated autonomic failure is multifactorial: pathophysiological mechanisms (hypoglycemia-associated autonomic failure) and factors of self-treatment behavior/self-management are crucial. For clinical use, simple diagnostic approaches (structured anamnesis, questionnaire tools, specific blood glucose levels, glucose monitoring) and effective treatment strategies are available. Decisive for the effective treatment of hypoglycemia problems is a multimodal approach that takes physiological factors, insulin therapy, and the self-management of patients equally into account and optimizes.

Introduction

The study results for the prognosis of type 1 and type 2 diabetes demonstrate the importance of a blood glucose adjustment that is as close to the norm as possible to prevent microangiopathic – possibly also macroangiopathic – complications.

As a result, a larger percentage of insulin-treated diabetes patients achieved significantly better glycemic control in the last decade.

However, the therapeutic goal of "normoglycemia" also increases the risk of hypoglycemia, which is increasingly becoming the focus of diabetes therapy as a limiting factor in insulin therapy. Proof of this is also the significant increase in scientific publications on this topic. According to MEDLINE research, the number of publications on the subject of hypoglycemia has increased by over 50% in the last 10 years. Due to the rapid increase in the number of diabetes patients who inject insulin – currently, at least 1.2 million insulin-treated diabetics are expected in Germany – a further increase in patients with hypoglycemia problems is to be expected.

Severe hypoglycemias have a high potential for self- or external danger. Especially in older age and in connection with concomitant diseases, severe hypoglycemia can pose a high health risk for people with diabetes and in extreme cases even end in death. In addition, hypoglycemia's intervened directly in the daily routine and require an interruption of the everyday routine for the treatment of hypoglycemia. The possibility or the real experience of suffering severe hypoglycemia and acting helplessly or uncontrollably in public can become an additional source of stress or even fear. It is therefore not surprising that hypoglycemia and its consequences are experienced by patients as one of the greater diabetes-related burdens and are associated with an increase in anxiety disorders and depressive illnesses.

Definition of hypoglycemia A uniform definition of hypoglycemia does not exist, which makes it difficult to compare the study results.

In the guidelines of the German Diabetes Society, hypoglycemia is defined as a blood glucose level < 50 mg/dl [2.8 mmol/l]. This blood glucose threshold is not without controversy in the literature. Due to the current knowledge regarding the pathophysiology of a disturbed hypoglycemia perception, a threshold value of blood glucose for the definition of hypoglycemia would be useful, which is above the symptom threshold of non-diabetics or diabetics with intact hypoglycemia perception. Therefore, the limit value proposed by the DDG appears to be too low, the blood glucose threshold proposed by Mühlhauser [17] < 60 mg/dl (3.4 mmol/l) for the definition of hypoglycemia appears more appropriate.

From a clinical point of view, hypoglycemia can also be divided according to its severity. "Mild" hypoglycemias are detected in time by the affected person and treated by fast-acting carbohydrates themselves. In the case of so-called "severe hypoglycemia", external help is required for treatment.

"Very severe hypoglycemia" requires glucose or glucagon injection as a result of the strong clouding of consciousness or unconsciousness. While very severe hypoglycemias treated by glucagon or glucose injection can be objectified based on prescriptions or doctor's reports, severe hypoglycemia (external help by supporting the consumption of fast-acting carbohydrates) is often difficult to verify the event. However, it is still useful to record severe hypoglycemia, as these can serve as risk markers for very severe hypoglycemia with unconsciousness, seizures, or a high hypoglycemia-related external or self-endangerment.

The frequency of hypoglycemia hypoglycemias is more or less unavoidable for people with type 1 diabetes who strive for a normal setting. In this group of patients, it can be assumed that there is at least two mild hypoglycemia per week.

A much more accurate estimate of the frequency of such mild hypoglycemia may be possible in the future with the help of continuous glucose measurement. Here, initial results show that the frequency of low blood glucose levels – especially at night – is much higher than the selective blood glucose controls suggest.

The frequency of severe hypoglycemia, for the treatment of which external assistance was necessary, was 0.64 per patient and year in intensified insulin therapy in the Diabetes Control and Complications Trial (DCCT); very severe hypoglycemia with unconsciousness or seizure was observed 0.19 times per patient per year. For Germany, the rates of very severe hypoglycemia in type 1 diabetics are between 0.16 and 0.28 per patient per year. Although the definition of very severe hypoglycemias used in German studies (glucose or glucagon injection required) differs slightly from the definition used in the DCCT (unconsciousness or seizure), there is a high degree of agreement between the German and US prevalence data.

In various studies, several risk factors have emerged that indicate an increased risk of hypoglycemia in type 1 diabetics. These include a low HbA1c value, previous hypoglycemia, reduced hypoglycemia perception, and lack of insulin residual secretion (negative C peptide). It can be assumed that about 20 - 30% of type 1 diabetes patients are affected by an increased risk of hypoglycemia.

A similar accumulation of severe hypoglycemias also seems to exist in type 2 diabetes. Henderson et al. report that severe hypoglycemia occurred in only 32 out of 215 types 2 diabetics (14.8%). However, there was also a subgroup of 7 patients in whom two or more severe hypoglycemia's occurred. Interestingly, in type 2 diabetes, the risk of severe hypoglycemia was not associated with a lower HbA1c value, but with higher age, a longer duration of diabetes, insulin treatment, and impaired hypoglycemia perception.

Causes of hypoglycemia problems for the occurrence of hypoglycemia problems, both physiological conditions, the core of which is an adaptation process to low blood sugar levels, and the self-management of those affected play a role.

Physiological conditions of hypoglycemia problems On the physiological side, a change in the blood glucose level, the so-called glycemic thresholds, from which a physiological reaction to the falling blood glucose level takes place, is an essential predisposing prerequisite for a disturbed hypoglycemia perception.

Normally, the human body is effectively protected from blood glucose drop by various hierarchically arranged physiological mechanisms.

The hierarchically arranged consequences of a low blood glucose level (activation of the autonomic nervous system, hormonal counter-regulation, neuroglycopenia) result in a treatment window in which effective self-treatment of hypoglycemia is possible. On the one hand, this treatment window is defined by the time or glycemic threshold from which the first symptoms (autonomic and neuroglycopenic warning symptoms) appear. On the other hand, the end of the time window is reached when neuroglycopenia becomes so severe (disorientation, clouding, or loss of consciousness) that effective self-treatment is no longer possible. Normally, the first hypoglycemia warning symptoms occur at glucose values between 50 mg/dl (2.8 mmol/l) and 55 mg/dl (3.1 mmol/l), while a loss of ability to act is usually only to be feared at glucose values of less than 35 mg/dl (1.9 mmol/l) so that a sufficiently large treatment window for effective self-treatment of low blood glucose results.

Unfortunately, type 1 diabetes leads to a loss of glucagon response to hypoglycemia after a longer period of diabetes. Another problem is that the other glycemic thresholds for hormonal counter-regulation and symptom response are not constant. Frequent, mild hypoglycemia can be used to adapt to low blood glucose levels, the exact mechanism of which is not yet fully understood. As a result, the protective hormonal counter-regulation and the warning symptoms only occur at lower blood glucose levels, and the "treatment window" between the first occurrence of warning symptoms and the onset of inability to act is reduced.

Cryer speaks in connection with this adjustment mechanism of a "Circulus Vitiosus" [18]. In this "vicious circle", a poorer perception of hypoglycemia causes an increase in low blood glucose levels, which further intensifies the adaptation process described above. Although this model was developed by Cryer and collaborators for type 1 diabetics, recent studies have shown that low blood glucose levels can also lead to an adjustment process in type 2 diabetics with a longer period of diabetes, which lowers the glycemic thresholds for the occurrence of warning symptoms and glucose back regulation. Thus, even in insulin-treated type 2 diabetics, after a longer period of diabetes and good glycemic control, an increased occurrence of hypoglycemia problems is to be expected.

Self-management and hypoglycemia problems

From a clinical perspective, the pathophysiological conditions of impaired hypoglycemia perception cannot be considered separately from self-treatment behavior. Such behavioral factors can include an accidental overdose of insulin, an incorrect assessment of the amount of insulin or the blood sugar efficacy of carbohydrates, as well as a lack of consideration of lifestyle habits such as physical activity or alcohol consumption. To influence these factors and to provide patients with the necessary skills for an adequate implementation of insulin therapy, intensive training of diabetics is necessary.

The behavioral causes of low blood glucose levels can also involve more or less stable attitudes and beliefs of the patient (so-called "health beliefs"). Such influencing factors include, for example, "over-averse" blood glucose target ranges and an overestimation of the individual risk of secondary diseases.

Hypoglycemia perception is often seen as a purely physiologically mediated process. However, recent studies show that in addition to the physiological conditions of a hypoglycemia perception, psychological factors can play a decisive role. Thus, the perception of body symptoms is not exclusively determined by their intensity, but also by the individual ability to accept and the degree of distraction or concentration on body processes. The recognition of certain symptoms as specific warning symptoms of hypoglycemia is also characterized by the knowledge of the patient, his previous experience with hypoglycemia, and his expectations. Also, the recognition of hypoglycemia symptoms does not necessarily lead to immediate treatment of hypoglycemia. For the speed with which a treatment decision is made about hypoglycemia, the individual willingness to take risks, the subjective importance of the activity currently being carried out, and the willingness to treat low blood glucose in public are decisive.

Modern treatment concepts for people with hypoglycemia problems, therefore, start from a bio-psychosocial perspective, in which the physiological conditions of hypoglycemia problems and the factors of self-management described above are equally taken into account. Cox's group has integrated these various somatic and psychological influencing factors into a biopsychosocial model of hypoglycemia management.

Diagnostic

Approaches for clinical practice, a variety of easy-to-use diagnostic strategies are available.

Specific diagnostic techniques, such as the use of portable small computers or artificial blood glucose manipulations (hypoglycemic clamps), are currently reserved for research purposes or narrowly defined questions in clinical applications.

Identification of high-risk patients The described risk factors for the occurrence of severe hypoglycemia and hypoglycemia problems are well suited for the early identification of high-risk patients and are relatively easy and unobtrusively accessible in medical documentation.

For this group of patients, further diagnostic measures or preventive interventions may be useful.

From a clinical point of view, when identifying high-risk patients, the risk potential that can emanate from hypoglycemia in certain patient groups must also be taken into account. This applies in particular to multimorbid or geriatric diabetes patients, for whom the prevention of hypoglycemia should be a high priority in the treatment or the field of pediatric diabetology.

Structured hypoglycemia history A decisive prerequisite for a valid anamnesis is the clarification of central terminology in conversation with the patients to avoid misunderstandings and misinformation.

For example, diabetes patients differ greatly in terms of their understanding of what is "mild" and "severe" hypoglycemia. Even terms such as "external help" often require a more precise explanation. It is also known that there are large interindividual differences in how one's hypoglycemia perceptibility is assessed – regardless of the actual hypoglycemia perception quality.

As a guideline for a structured hypoglycemia history, the questionnaire developed by Clarke and colleagues is well suited. In addition to the evaluation mode described by the authors (dichotomous result: "intact" vs. impaired hypoglycemia perception), a qualitative consideration of the instrument may also be useful in clinical practice (e.B. change in glycemic thresholds for hypoglycemia symptoms). This must be supplemented by a detailed dialectological history including a reconstruction of the causes of any (severe) hypoglycemia, B such as dysfunctional insulin therapy or errors in self-treatment.

Evaluation: Each ticked, italicized field is counted as one point. Question 3 and 4: In the case of the frequency of severe hypoglycemia, a number 0 than one point each is evaluated. Questions 5 and 6: A point is awarded if the frequency of asymptomatic hypoglycemia (question 6) is greater than that of hypoglycemias with symptoms (question 5). The points achieve are summed up. An overall score greater than two is counted as the presence of a hypoglycemia perception problem.

It is also important to ask about individual attitudes towards hypoglycemia, such as fears of hypoglycemia and secondary diseases, blood glucose target values, and the acceptance of short-term elevated blood glucose levels or the usual treatment of hypoglycemia.

Standardized questionnaires in addition to an in-depth history of hypoglycemia, the use of standardized and validated psychometric instruments makes sense for patients with hypoglycemia problems.

Thus, e.B. the perception of hypoglycemia and hypoglycemia-associated emotional stresses, such as the fear of hypoglycemia, can be recorded in a standardized manner. In addition, hypoglycemia nonspecific questionnaire methods exist, which are also suitable for screening for hypoglycemia problems.

Building on the Edinburgh Hypoglycemia Scale, McAulay and colleagues propose a symptom checklist for clinical use to record individual hypoglycemia symptoms. The patients are given this checklist with the instruction to mark which of the listed hypoglycemia symptoms they typically feel or on which signs they recognize hypoglycemia (or during hypoglycemia, which symptoms they are currently experiencing). This enables a quick overview of individual symptom profiles and intensities and can provide additional indications of a hypoglycemia perception problem, e.g. in the characteristic absence of autonomous hypoglycemia symptoms. This questionnaire is also well suited for follow-up and review of the effects of therapeutic measures on hypoglycemia perception. In addition, the authors recommend that an additional item assess and document the hypoglycemia perception ability of the patients on a seven-point scale (from "very good" to "very bad") ("How good is my hypoglycemia perception?").

It should be borne in mind that this checklist is an instrument developed for diabetes patients in adulthood. There are systematic differences between the listed symptoms and signs of hypoglycemia, which often occur in children or geriatric diabetes patients, which are partly due to the interception and verbalization abilities of these patient groups. In childhood, for example, behavioral symptoms of hypoglycemia are more common (e.B irrational and "over-the-top" behavior, and neurological symptoms sometimes come to the fore in elderly or geriatric patients. More non-specific symptoms (e.B. weakness) are often not attributed to hypoglycemia but are otherwise attributed. These peculiarities should be taken into account when assessing hypoglycemia perception and the survey of hypoglycemia symptoms. A symptom checklist adapted for elderly patients is also available.

The most established instrument for recording fears of hypoglycemia is the Hypoglycemia Fear Survey in its revised version (HFS-R). This questionnaire contains two subscales that measure the cognitive level ("worry" scale; Concern about hypoglycemia) or the behavioral level of hypoglycemia anxiety ("behavior" scale; e.g. items on avoidance behavior, B.dem such as intentionally "raising" the blood sugar level).

The German-language hypoglycemia anxiety inventory (HAI), on the other hand, enables a differentiated recording of hypoglycemia-related fears (cognitive, emotional, and behavioral level) in clinical use and is suitable against this background to derive initial indications for therapeutic measures in this regard.

In addition to the described hypoglycemia-specific survey instruments, further questionnaires may be useful in clinical practice. One example is the Problem Areas in Diabetes Questionnaire (PAID). This instrument uses a total of 20 items to record different potential (emotional) problem areas and diabetes-specific burdens, including the burden of hypoglycemia. The instrument is well suited as a screening instrument in clinical applications and enables the rapid identification of patients with diabetes-specific burdens. It is also used by the Joslin Diabetes Center as a standard screening for all patients. A German-language version and tentative standard values for Germany are available.

Another useful tool is the therapy satisfaction questionnaire by Clare Bradley (Diabetes Treatment Satisfaction Questionnaire, DTSQ), which records therapy satisfaction across a total of eight items. This instrument has established itself internationally for recording therapy satisfaction (e.g. to check the effects of therapy changes or training measures) and contains an additional item for recording the subjectively experienced frequency of hypoglycemia, which can be used as an indicator of corresponding experiences due to hypoglycemia.

Exposure to low blood glucose levels from a pathophysiological perspective, exposure to low blood glucose levels is of crucial importance in the genesis of impaired hypoglycemia awareness.

Against this background, Kvetched and his colleagues introduced the so-called Low Blood Glucose Index (LBGI) as a risk indicator for the occurrence of severe hypoglycemia. Through a logarithmic transformation, low blood glucose levels are weighted more heavily. The authors were able to show that the predictive value of this LBGI exceeds that of HbA1c about future severe hypoglycemia and, together with the risk factor, elucidates severe hypoglycemia in the anamnesis, 40% of the variance. Similarly, it could also be shown that the percentage of low measured values (< 60 mg/dl or 3.3 mmol/l) in the total number of measurements makes a significant contribution to the prediction of the occurrence of severe hypoglycemia. A disadvantage of such an approach is that the data quality is decisively influenced by the self-control frequency or. deem individual self-control behavior).

Although the analysis of the blood glucose values documented by the patients already offers the possibility of calculating corresponding characteristic values, measuring devices with a comprehensive storage function, in particular, allow easier access and the transfer of the data to a PC. This means that the clinical user has the opportunity to calculate parameters such as the LBGI more easily. This procedure also has the advantage that by the use of measuring instruments with memory function to compared to the logged self-control values more objective data is recurred.

Glucose tracking for some time now, structures for medical software were available in Germany that permits non-stop monitoring of glucose.

In principle, the continuous registration of glucose has the advantage over conventional point measurement that short-term glycemic excursions can be detected that would otherwise remain undetected: in principle, the continuous measurement allows a complete and thus more valid detection of hypoglycemic glucose derailments and exposure to low glucose levels. This makes the use of glucose monitoring particularly interesting in patients with frequent and/or asymptomatic hypoglycemia. There are currently two systems available in Germany for continuous glucose measurement, the Continuous Glucose Monitoring System (GCMS, Medtronic Minimed) and the GlucoDay system (Menarini Diagnostics), which can be classified as good in terms of clinical accuracy (for exact specifications of the systems see). These systems allow monitoring for a maximum of 72 (GCMS) or 48 (GlucoDay) hours and provide a measured value every five or three minutes.

It should be borne in mind, however, that the systems currently available monitor the interstitial glucose content - the exact relationship to blood glucose, especially in the case of rapid blood glucose waste and increases, has not yet been clarified. Recently, there have also been some studies that critically question the measurement accuracy in the hypoglycemic range (e.B. the problem of "flat-lining" or the registration of prolonged hypoglycemic episodes with the GCMS that do not correspond to the actual glucose course).

About the clinical benefits of monitoring in patients with hypoglycemia problems, the study situation is very limited, but some of the results are promising. In some smaller studies, it was clearly shown that the use of continuous monitoring increased the detection rate, reduced the incidence of biochemical hypoglycemia, and stabilized glycemic control. Especially in patients with hypoglycemia perception problems or for the detection of undetected hypoglycemia, monitoring can be helpful.

Another theoretically interesting application is the use of a glucose monitor as a "warning system", i.e. a monitor that warns the patient of impending hypoglycemia using a corresponding signal. In contrast to the GCMS, the GlucoDay system has a "warning function", i.e. a hypo- or hyperglycemic threshold can be set by the user, from which the device can alert the patient by acoustic and/or vibration signals. However, there are no studies to date in which this function and its clinical benefits have been systematically investigated. It should also be pointed out that neither of the two monitoring systems is a patient system. Rather, they are expert systems, i.e. the devices are designed to be used by the practitioner as a diagnostic instrument - and not for use in everyday life by the patients.

Further diagnostic approaches Portable small computers ("handheld computers", e.B. on the technical basis of a commercially available organizer) are often used as "electronic diary" for research purposes.

This offers the methodological advantage that data can be collected more objectively as well as more time-related and thus closer to everyday life than via conventional paper-and-pencil protocols, which facilitates the analysis and evaluation of the data. Such systems are also used in research in the field of diabetes. It remains to be seen how blood glucose meters/software that offer similar possibilities (e.B. OneTouch Ultra smart / Life scan; Pocket Compass / Roche), in clinical practice.

Experimental hypoglycemia inductions by hyperinsulinemia clamps as a further possibility of apparatus diagnostics for hypoglycemia problems do not represent a standard diagnosis for clinical practice but are reserved for special questions (e.B. quantification of counter-regulation, endocrinological questions).

Therapeutic approaches for hypoglycemia problems Due to the multifactorial genesis of hypoglycemia problems, the therapy should be aimed both at optimizing insulin therapy to reduce the frequency of hypoglycemia, improving hypoglycemia perception, and optimizing the patient's self-management to improve the handling of hypoglycemia.

In addition to a possible modification of insulin therapy, an improvement of the self-treatment behavior through general (e.B. repetition training) or special training measures (e.B. systematic hypoglycemia perception training) is often useful. For special problems in connection with hypoglycemia (e.B. hypoglycemia anxiety), the use of psychotherapeutic strategies can be helpful. By the results of the diagnosis, the severity of the hypoglycemia problem as well as the psychosocial consequences for the patient (e.B. loss of driving license, professional difficulties, loss of quality of life), the following therapy strategies have proven themselves in clinical practice.

Systematic analysis of previous hypoglycemia's in every discussion of blood glucose levels, should be systematically recorded whether, how often, and due to which causes hypoglycemia has occurred.

At the knowledge level, it must be checked whether the patient has sufficient knowledge about insulin therapy, possible causes of hypoglycemia, and the effect of insulin correction measures. In the event of hypoglycemia, it should be systematically considered together with the patient whether the insulin dosage (or the dosage of insulin tropic drugs) was too high, occurred at the wrong time or whether the insulin strategy should be reconsidered, whether hypoglycemia's occurred due to errors in insulin dosage/injection or was caused by a lack of consideration of altered insulin sensitivity (e.B. due to weight reduction, increased physical fitness, improved blood glucose levels). Too low intake of carbohydrates (e.B. due to an exuberant meal, estimation errors, diarrhea, vomiting), physical activity without adequate reduction in insulin dosage and/or without increased carbohydrate intake or alcohol consumption without appropriate precautions are also common causes of hypoglycemia, which can be justified by errors in self-treatment.

In the analysis of the causes of hypoglycemia, possible concomitant diseases (e.B. gastroparesis, reduced renal insulin clearance, increased glucose consumption as a result of extrapancreatic tumors, disorders of gluconeogenesis due to liver/kidney diseases, endocrinopathies, alcoholism, malnutrition) should also be taken into account, which often leads to a significantly increased risk of severe hypoglycemia. For these patients, the avoidance of hypoglycemia is a very important therapeutic goal, special training measures for the prevention of hypoglycemia are recommended. This also applies to patients in whom signs of hypoglycemia are caused by concomitant medication or are masked in their symptoms (e.B. sedative medication, antihypertensive drugs).

Optimization of insulin therapy If the analysis of insulin therapy reveals possible causes of hypoglycemia problems (e.B. un physiological basal insulin supply, overlapping insulin bolus, circadian fluctuations in insulin sensitivity, difficult to predict insulin absorption courses), a change in the current therapy regimen (e.B. change in the basal insulin content, BE factors) or the use of "physiological" forms of therapy (intensified insulin therapy, insulin pump therapy, if necessary insulin analogs) should be considered in these patients.

The use of insulin analogs can be a helpful option to reduce the number of hypoglycemia, despite still not being studied on this topic. As a further option, insulin pump therapy (CSII) can bring benefits for the reduction of hypoglycemia. In a recent meta-analysis of a total of twelve randomized controlled studies on the effectiveness of CSII, a significant reduction in blood glucose variability in the sense of fluctuations was demonstrated in addition to an improvement in HbA1c by an average of 0.56%. However, it should be borne in mind that due to the heterogeneity of the study designs included in the meta-analysis, no valid statements can be made about the effects of CSII on the frequency of hypoglycemia.

After severe hypoglycemia, the patient should strive for the strict avoidance of further hypoglycemia, since even single hypoglycemia can significantly reduce the counter-regulation in the event of further hypoglycemia. In patients with hypoglycemia unawareness, the avoidance of hypoglycemia ("scrupulous avoidance of hypoglycemia"), is an important strategy to normalize hypoglycemia perception. This is reversible, even if the hormonal counter-regulation does not return to fully normal. With consistent avoidance of - even mild and particularly nocturnal hypoglycemia - a significant improvement in hypoglycemia perception can occur in these patients after only 2-3 weeks. To achieve this, a modification of the blood glucose target values and an increase in the blood glucose test frequency is usually recommended. Higher blood glucose target values are particularly useful for avoiding nocturnal hypoglycemia. However, this can be accompanied by an increase in the HbA1c value and must be discussed and determined together with the patient, taking into account any existing diabetic sequelae.

Modification of dysfunctional attitudes in the search for the causes of hypoglycemia, the personal attitudes and beliefs of the patient (so-called "health beliefs") in connection with hypoglycemia should also be addressed.

Hypoglycemia problems are often due to overly "ambitious" blood glucose target values, which result either from concern about possible complications of diabetes or from a careless attitude towards possible risks due to hypoglycemia. To record possible dysfunctional attitudes, the following areas should be addressed: Targeted HbA1c target value, targeted blood glucose target range at night, assessments of one's own risk of secondary diseases and hypoglycemia, fear of hypoglycemia or subsequent complications, individual "feel-good area" about blood glucose values. If the glycemic target areas sought by the patient represent a cause of recurrent hypoglycemia and/or hypoglycemia problems, these should be discussed with the patient and modified if possible.

Optimization of self-treatment behavior to avoid hypoglycemia Since hypoglycemia is mainly caused by errors in self-treatment, strategies should be developed for recurrent hypoglycemia as part of special, problem-related training with the patient to improve the handling of hypoglycemia.

Here, a detailed analysis of the individual insulin active profiles is carried out with the patient. Based on the previous hypoglycemia history, specific risk situations (e.B. nocturnal hypoglycemias, sports) are identified, prospective treatment strategies for early risk minimization (e.B. determination of glycemic target values for certain situations, blood glucose test frequency) are defined and automated treatment routines, as well as adequate treatment measures (e.B. correction rules, availability of "Hypo-BE"), are developed and practically practiced. Corresponding curricula, training materials, and patient documents, which were developed and evaluated by cox's working group, among others, are also available in a German translation.

Optimization of the treatment behavior in hypoglycemia Through suitable training measures, the behavior in hypoglycemia can also be optimized. These include strategies for systematically directing attention to the body's warning signs, developing routine "check-ups" to identify specific symptoms of hypoglycemia, developing treatment routines (e.B.g. "eat first, then measure"), and defining measures to facilitate the rapid availability and intake of Hypo-BE for the patient. In the case of hypoglycemia perception disorders, which are associated with a loss of internal warning signals, the targeted inclusion of external stimuli for an impending risk of hypoglycemia is particularly important. These include measures such as an increased self-control frequency, the calculation of estimating variables for a future hypoglycemia risk, or the targeted involvement of other people (external perception by relatives, friends, professional colleagues). Likewise, treatment barriers that occur in hypoglycemia (e.B. conflicts with the partner) can be analyzed and adaptive strategies developed. The inclusion of relatives in the training is therefore very useful, not least because of the high burden that relatives experience due to the hypoglycemia of the partner. In the case of particularly vulnerable persons (e.B. persons living alone, patients with psychiatric comorbidity), it is advisable to draw up a concrete emergency plan to ensure the availability of rapid assistance.

Systematic training of hypoglycemia perception Results of experimental intervention research proves on the one hand that the interoceptive perception of cues of hypoglycemia is subject to errors and distortions since these do not take place independently of feelings, thoughts, and memories.

On the other hand, they also show that interoceptive sensory perception can be improved. Based on these findings, the working group led by Daniel J. Cox developed a structured perception training for better detection of hypo- and hyperglycemic blood glucose levels (Blood Glucose Awareness Training, BGAT, German translation). For this purpose, there is evidence of efficacy about the reduction of severe hypoglycemia, improved hypoglycemia perception, improved glycemic control, an increase in knowledge about hypoglycemia, the improvement of adrenaline response to a hypoglycemic stimulus, and the reduction of hypoglycemia-related traffic problems.

A prerequisite for better recognition of symptoms is systematic introspection. Keeping a "hypo-diary" and using special symptom lists makes it possible to detect warnings for hypoglycemia and to identify the reliable and early symptoms. Patients are instructed to estimate the current blood sugar before the measurement with any suspicion of hypoglycemia, if necessary also with each blood glucose measurement, to observe all possible symptoms and to note abnormalities. The systematic evaluation of such a diary provides answers to the question of which symptoms are particularly reliable in indicating hypoglycemia. Likewise, both patients and practitioners receive feedback about the actual hypoglycemia perception quality.

Since the nature and intensity of hypoglycemia warning symptoms often change with increasing duration, patients with perception problems, in particular, should recognize that their symptom pattern has changed over the years. It is known that when the thresholds shift, the autonomic symptoms are particularly affected, which often occur very late or not at all so that the patient is now forced to concentrate more on the neuroglycopenic symptoms. In contrast to the autonomic symptoms, however, the neuroglycopenic symptoms are often much harder to recognize. In addition, advanced neuroglycopenia can limit the patient's ability to perceive and act. It is therefore advisable to specifically train the perception of neuroglycopenic symptoms in a targeted manner. For this purpose, a series of exercises are available, with the help of which the perceptual ability of interoceptive cues can be improved.

Reduction of psychosocial stress due to hypoglycemia Since recurrent hypoglycemia can lead to psychosocial stress, reduced quality of life, depressive moods, and anxiety, psychotherapeutic support should be offered to patients with increased stress due to hypoglycemia or an increased risk of developing a manifest mental illness.

For patients with hypoglycemia anxiety, several psychotherapeutic treatment measures are also available.

Conclusion for practice The risk of hypoglycemia increases the closer to norm a blood glucose adjustment takes place: Hypoglycemia problems are a decisive limiting factor for the therapeutic goal normoglycemia.

The prevalence of hypoglycemia problems in type 1 diabetes patients is 20-30%. The data on the situation in type 2 diabetes are still inconsistent, but recent studies suggest that insulin-dependent type 2 diabetes patients may also be affected by hypoglycemia problems. Risk groups can be identified by parameters that are very easy to collect in clinical practice so that appropriate preventive measures can be initiated. Simple diagnostic strategies and procedures are available that capture both the pathophysiological level of hypoglycemia problems (exposure to low blood glucose levels) and factors of self-treatment behavior and "health beliefs". To effectively treat hypoglycemia problems, first of all, attention should be paid to the prevention of hypoglycemia. For this purpose, it is crucial to optimize both insulin therapy and the self-treatment behavior of the patients. Problem-specific training and treatment concepts have proven themselves in the treatment of hypoglycemia problems and should be made accessible to every affected patient.

Running in comparison with heavy physical exertion for the prevention of cardiovascular events in women

In the prevention of cardiovascular diseases, the importance of running compared to heavy physical exertion is controversially discussed. In particular, there is little data for women from ethnic or racial minority groups.

Methods:

Prospectively, the overall physical activity score, running, heavy physical exertion, and hours spent sitting were examined as predictors of the incidence of coronary events as well as all cardiovascular events in 73,743 postmenopausal women between the ages of 50 and 79 in the Women's Health Initiative Observational

Study. At the beginning of the study, the participants had neither a diagnosed cardiovascular disease nor cancer and completed a detailed questionnaire on physical activity.

Results:

345 newly diagnosed cases of coronary heart disease and a total of 1,551 cardiovascular events were documented.

An increasing physical activity score showed a strong inverse association with the risk of both coronary events and cardiovascular events as a whole. Similar results were found for white women of color. Women with increasing quintiles for energy consumption – measured in metabolic equivalents (MET score) – had an age-adjusted relative risk for coronary events of 1.00, 0.73, 0.69, 0.68, and 0.47 respectively ($p<0.001$ for the trend). In multivariate analyses, the strong inverse relationship between the total MET score and the risk of cardiovascular events remained (respective adjusted relative risks for increasing quintiles: 1.00, 0.89, 0.81, 0.78, and 0.72; $p < 0.001$ for the trend). Running and strong physical activity was associated with similar risk reductions, and the results did not differ fundamentally by race, age, or body mass index. In addition, a researcher running speed and fewer sedentary hours a day predicted a lower risk.

Conclusion:

These prospective data indicate that both walking and heavy physical activity are associated with significant reductions in the incidence of cardiovascular events in postmenopausal women, regardless of race, ethnicity, age, and body mass index. Extensive sitting predicts an increased cardiovascular risk.

Comment:

Women with diabetes represent a special risk group for cardiovascular events and should therefore be particularly motivated to engage in physical activity. It should be noted that increased physical activity, regardless of weight loss, already leads to a significant improvement in mortality.

"Fat burner" sports

Fitness is on everyone's lips. Fitness is booming. But how do you manage to become "really fit" and, if possible, to stay fit? Take a healthy path to more physical fitness and well-being with diabetes.

Many diets fail because an important building block is missing: regular endurance training. It does not come down to sweaty peak performance: Training in the middle pulse range (fat burning zone) helps to reduce annoying pounds effectively and permanently.

Training in the optimal pulse range No matter whether you cycle, swim or walk: Your pulse should be in the individual fat-burning range.

At the beginning of training, you mainly burn carbohydrates. After about 20 to 30 minutes, the body switches to fat burning. However, only if you stay in your fat-burning zone. Three to four times a week at least half an hour of training is optimal to boost fat burning. If you are a fitness beginner, start with three times

10 minutes a week. Only encourage yourself to do as much as you can in the long run. Exercise not only helps with weight loss, but it also brings fun, relaxes, and has a positive effect on blood sugar.

Swimming

In the water, you only feel ten percent of your actual body weight. Therefore, swimming is a joint-friendly fat burner training. It is particularly suitable for fitness beginners, heavily overweight people, and water rats. When swimming, not only do pounds melt in the long term, but you increase your endurance, mobility, and sense of balance. Variety in the swimming style works more effectively: a track chest, a track crawl, and a trackback swim. To prevent tension in the neck area, strive for a flat swimming position when breaststroke. The head is half in the water. With knee problems, crawling and back swimming are more relieving.

Walking and Nordic Walking

Walking is less strenuous than jogging. If you are overweight by more than six kilos, you should walk instead of jog. It protects your joints, because here - unlike jogging - the flight phase is missing, as always afoot remains in contact with the ground. Walking is possible not only outdoors, but also on a treadmill in the gym or at home. Another type of walking is Nordic walking. It is dynamic walking with specially designed poles, similar to cross-country skiing. A comparison with normal walking showed that up to 45 percent more calories are burned at the same speed. Walking and Nordic walking are optimal fat burner sports that help you to keep your weight under control in the long term. Do not forget about stretching before and after training: this is how to avoid muscle strains and shortening the ligaments. When walking, pay attention to shoes that give you a firm hold and leave enough space for the foot. To help you find the right shoes, let us advise you in a sports shop.

Cycling

The bike is an optimal fat burner. When cycling, you train endurance and a sense of balance. You quickly feel physical success, and your condition improves enormously. If you prefer indoor training, you can achieve equally good results in the gym or on an exercise bike. To avoid accidents, a cycling helmet and tight-fitting sports trousers padded on the buttocks are recommended.

Regular training brings it Through regular training, you permanently increase your physical basal metabolic rate and burn more energy - even in resting phases.

If you like to practise different sports, your body will be all the more pleased. Variety in training makes fat deposits melt more easily.

EATING DISORDERS: CONSULTANTS AND DOCTORS ARE IMPORTANT MEDIATORS

Eating disorders in people with diabetes are experienced again and again by consultants and doctors in practice. Insulin therapy of patients is often very difficult. It is characterized by strongly fluctuating blood glucose values with pronounced hyper- or hypoglycemias. Patients come to the practice or clinic to have "their sugar" adjusted. However, a good blood sugar adjustment is usually only possible if the eating disorder has been treated beforehand. Diabetes consultants and doctors play an important role as the first contact person and mediator.

The most important psychosomatic eating disorders include anorexia nervosa and bulimia nervosa. In addition, there are a large number of unspecified eating disorders or atypical forms. The quantity of sufferers has risen gradually in recent years. The figures for anorexia nervosa vary between 4.2 and 8.2 per 100,000 inhabitants. Between the ages of 15 and 19, the incidence rate rises to 56.7 per 100,000 inhabitants. The prevalence of bulimia nervosa in young women is 2 to 4.5%. These diseases affect more women than men (5 to 10% of all disturbed eaters), although the proportion of men has increased in recent years. The prevalence of bulimia nervosa is higher in type 1 diabetics compared to anorexia nervosa and can be up to 3%. The prevalence of unspecified eating disorders is significantly increased.

In most cases, eating disorders have clear comorbidity to depressive disorders. Mortality is significantly increased in type 1 diabetics with anorexia nervosa, and the risk of retinopathy is tripled in patients with type 2 and bulimia nervosa.

Slimming mania as a cause?

The idealized beauty picture is considered a cause of eating disorders. However, people with diabetes often also give as a reason that they perceive food as compulsive ("diet cycle"), they reject this "need to eat". Often, diabetes itself is not accepted.

These reasons cannot be held solely responsible. The causes often lie in a fundamental conflict in the search for one's own identity or the struggle between dependence and self-determination. Often there is an extremely close parent-child relationship. An eating disorder usually begins between the ages of 14 and 25 years.

Anorexia nervosa (anorexia nervosa) is an eating disorder in which those affected strive for minimum body weight (BMI < 17 kg/m2). The perception of figure, weight, and appearance is disturbed. In addition, there is often depression and social isolation. Anorexia, as a rule, develops during puberty as a struggle for demarcation against the parents.

The problems that exist in anorectic patients with insulin therapy are mainly in estimating the need for insulin. Due to the very low body weight, hypoglycemia can easily develop due to an incorrectly estimated dose of insulin. Another problem can occur due to self-induced hyperglycemia: patients often omitted insulin injections before meals in order not to absorb the nutrients from the food (increase in glucosuria) and thus to be able to control the weight. This behavior can lead to ketoacidosis derailment. Anorectic patients often come to the practice and clinic with strongly fluctuating blood glucose values, with hypo problems or a derailment. In the hospital (and under controlled conditions), blood sugar can usually be adjusted to some extent. At home, however, the usual fluctuations occur again, as the causal problem is not resolved. Good blood sugar control can only be achieved when the cause, the eating disorder, has been treated. Patients need expert help for this, as the causes are very often to be sought in deeper conflicts. As diabetes and nutritionists, we can only act as mediators of the first contact between patient and psychologist.

Example of a patient with anorexia nervosa The patient has had type 1 diabetes mellitus for eleven years and has been treated with insulin pump therapy with Humalog for two years.

Hypoglycemias are experienced daily at values around 30 mg/dl with mostly reliable perception. Blood sugar fluctuations with daily hypoglycemia under a known anorexia nervosa (BMI 16 kg/m2) led to hospital admission. Furthermore, when ingested, there was also depressive symptomatology with anxiety.

Therapy: Because of her mental illness, the patient was regularly treated in our psychosocial department, and a psychiatric contact was also arranged with a registered psychiatrist. During inpatient treatment, a fundamental revision of the insulin dose took place. After successful correction adjustment, very good normoglycemic values were recently shown, at the same time hypoglycemia could be avoided with a few exceptions. Through insulin pump therapy, the patient can react as flexibly as possible to fluctuating food intake.

Diagnostic criteria
- Underweight (at least 15 % below the expected weight)
- Fear of weight gain
- Distorted body perception (own very low weight threshold)
- In women: amenorrhea
-   Weight loss is self-induced (avoidance of high-calorie foods, self-induced vomiting or dissipation, excessive physical activity, use of appetite suppressants and diuretics)
- In diabetes: unexplained blood sugar fluctuations and haggling over any insulin unit (IE)
Usually significantly increased HbA1cvalues

Bulimia nervosa (eating vomiting) is an eating disorder characterized by the alternation of eating attacks and attempts at weight loss. Typical here is a total loss of control in these seizures. As countermeasures, vomiting is usually carried out or laxatives and diuretics are misused. People with diabetes often simply leave out insulin as a countermeasure to the eating attacks. In this way, they avoid the absorption of nutrients (and thus the supposed weight gains).

Diagnostic criteria

- Feeding attacks
- Loss of control
- Weight loss is self-induced (self-induced vomiting or dissipation, exaggerated physical activity, use of appetite suppressants, diuretics, temporary periods of starvation, neglect of insulin therapy)
- Frequency of eating attacks
- Distorted body scheme
- Constant preoccupation with food
- In diabetes: inexplicably fluctuating blood glucose levels

The frequency of bulimia is relatively high in diabetics. In a psychosomatic clinic, 5 to 25% of bulimia patients are usually typing 1 diabetic.

In contrast to anorexia, those affected are well aware of their illness. This exerts enormous suffering pressure on the patients: they are often depressed and suicidal. In women with bulimia, there is very often an inner conflict between the desire to meet all external requirements perfectly and their own needs. Emerging conflicts are carried out in the form of eating-vomiting seizures.

The problems with insulin therapy are mainly to correctly assess the insulin requirement between the attacks of hunger and eating, and in the prevention of hyperglycemia as a result of the suspension of the insulin dose.

Example of two patients with bulimia nervosa at the age of 14, Ms. M. was diagnosed with type 1 diabetes mellitus.

Weight at manifestation was 56 kg at 1.68 m, their maximum weight was 70 kg. The therapy was initially conducted rather strictly. 8 meals/day was prescribed. The food bans on the one hand and the "need to eat" with hypoglycemia on the other hand made her enormous problems from the beginning. Although it has little to do with hypoglycemia, it still makes her angry when she "has to eat" in hypoglycemias. An optimal ICT has never been conducted before, blood glucose self-checks are carried out only very irregularly. Mrs. M. always squirts for feeling. There are always phases in which the patient does not apply insulin. The last HbA1c value was 15%. This fact, too, did not move the patient in any way to change anything. She simply accepted the value and "went on like this".

The eating disorder has been known to the patient for about 10 years, but it has developed insidiously. The triggers are diabetes mellitus, as well as the divorce of the parents. In 2000, the patient was in psychosomatic treatment, which lasted 3 months; since September 2001 she has been in outpatient care.

Therapy: It has now been switched to the long-acting insulin analog glargine (Lantus) before the night. Among these, the blood glucose levels could be significantly reduced. This insulin should relieve the therapy. The patient was trained on insulin therapy that was as flexible as possible without "dietary regulations". In addition, she was closely psychologically cared for by our psychosocial department. Ms. M. under patient treatment in a psychosomatic clinic immediately after discharge.

Mrs. K. was admitted because she had blood sugar derailments with last measured fasting values of 250 to 320 mg/dl in a known eating disorder (bulimia). The BMI is currently at 29 kg/m2. The manifestation of type 2 diabetes was detected during pregnancy 17 years ago. Most recently, insulin therapy ICT was carried out with Lantus at night and Humalog at meals with a daily insulin requirement of about 90-100 units. Metformin 850 mg is used in the morning and the evening. Hypoglycemia has not been experienced so far.

Therapy: There was care by the psychosocial department in the house, and further outpatient care was provided at home. The patient switched to a flexible ICT with Humalog and Protaphan at night. The amount of insulin could be significantly reduced to make it easier for the patient to lose weight.

Process standards of the ADDK It is important for diabetics with an eating disorder that the patients are treated and advised in a diabetes center with a medical and psychological care structure.

Here, a disorder-specific anamnesis and diagnosis must be carefully carried out. Furthermore, in the motivation phase, a psychotherapeutic further treatment should be prepared. The team of psychologists, doctors, and diabetes consultants can work together with the patient to develop a therapy regimen that is as variable as possible, which enables flexible eating behavior about the amount and times of food as well as the variety of foods.

Conclusion

Many patients with an eating disorder come to the clinic or practice to have their blood sugar adjusted. As a prerequisite for diabetes therapy, however, the therapy of the eating disorder is first necessary. Without this, the prognosis is extremely unfavorable and success rather unlikely. For this, however, the patient's insight is a prerequisite. Here, the consultant plays a decisive role as an intermediary. To be able to do justice to this role, no strict diabetes therapy should be chosen. The aim is to adjust the patient as flexibly as possible to his eating behavior, i.e. good basic care with flexible bolus administration. However, to be able to guarantee lasting success, it is above all important to treat the cause – the eating disorder – and this requires psychological help. First of all, in collaboration with an outpatient psychologist, therapy should be created. Optimal is a treatment in an appropriate psychosomatic institution. Contact addresses can be found on the Internet. Self-help groups for eating disorders are also located in almost every major city.

Relatives – (not) a topic?! - Mastering diabetes together

Diabetes not only affects people with diabetes themselves but usually has a variety of effects on the partnership, family, and other social relationships. Therefore, good management of diabetes is a joint task of relatives and the person affected.

"What do you need to be happy?" Researchers asked thousands of people in almost every country of the world in a large international study on the subject of quality of life. The result was astounding: whether rich or poor, regardless of ethnicity, skin color, or religion, the respondents named "health" as the most important prerequisite for happiness.

The second most important area was "to be socially integrated", to have a "harmonious family life and/or a good partnership" and to receive sufficient "social support from others".

Good support helps to cope better with diabetes The success of diabetes therapy depends crucially on whether the person concerned succeeds in taking care of his or her diabetes enough in everyday life.

It is, therefore, reasonable to assume that good support from others - partners, children, relatives, friends - can be very helpful for the successful management of diabetes, while a lack of support is an additional complication.

Several scientific studies confirm this connection. They show that the attitude to diabetes as well as the concrete blood sugar setting also depends on whether the person concerned receives satisfactory support from partners, family, or friends.

People with diabetes, who cope with their disease rather poorly and have a worse metabolic attitude, usually describe significantly worse support or less satisfying social relationships.

On the other hand, "health" is such an important life goal that the illness of a family member or partner naturally also strongly influences the lives of the relatives.

Relatives are also affected This is often not sufficiently taken into account. A child's diabetes disease affects the whole family - parents, siblings, grandparents alike. Of course, dealing with the daily therapy requirements also affects the everyday life of the rest of the family. Worries about possible hypoglycemia or blood sugar derailments as well as the occurrence of secondary diseases occupy relatives such as the affected person himself. In discussions on this subject, I have often noticed how relatives have spoken of "our" diabetes, which means nothing other than that the management of diabetes is seen as a common cause.

"I wouldn't have made it alone" Mr. Momsen was one of the first type 1 diabetics to be treated with insulin in Germany.

He lived with his illness for over 70 years without any significant complications. In a panel discussion, he answered my question as to what recommendation he would give other people with diabetes for successful handling of the disease: "Without my wife and children, I might by no means have been capable of trying this. As a diabetic, you depend on the support of your family. This is extremely important. Mastering the ups and downs of life together is what makes a good relationship. In other areas of life, of course, I was also able to support my wife and children. But I'm sure I wouldn't have had enough strength on my own to cope so well with the disease."

Family and partner relationships are particularly important Results of family research and family therapy clearly show that the family and a close partner relationship play a prominent role in social support.

For the most part, the family is the place where you can experience the most intense security, closeness, and intense affection. This is a very beneficial condition, especially for emotional coping with diabetes. Family security is especially important for men, as they usually have more difficulty showing feelings and therefore experience much less emotional support outside the family.

Good support - good against stress?

It is also known from stress research that, especially in the case of severe stress and crises, good support from others represents a kind of "buffer" against these stresses: for example, in the case of the occurrence of diabetes, severe hypoglycemia, or when dealing with subsequent complications.

Talking to someone else, exchanging feelings, experiencing physical contact, or simply feeling the closeness of the other can help to ensure that the perceived stress or strain does not exceed a certain extent. However, you have to take care of a good relationship with others at an early stage so that it is sustainable enough in difficult situations.

Support can be experienced positively as well as negatively Social support by others, however, is a double-edged sword: mostly it is experienced positively and as a support for life with diabetes; on the other hand, too much support or a false form of support can also have negative effects. This can be the case, for example, if overprotection and interference in the privacy of the individual hinder the self-reliant handling of diabetes. Adolescents with diabetes describe this as a common problem. Even too much concern for the partner can lead to the fact that the partner experiences this not as a support, but as a restriction and reacts with defense and withdrawal.

"Only you alone can do it, but you can't do it alone!"

This slogan of a self-help group expresses very well that the handling of the disease diabetes is of course first of all the thing of each

individual. But without good support from others, it is very difficult to cope well with diabetes in the long term; however, it does not fall from the sky but is the result of one's own efforts to cultivate friendships, to strive for a good, lively partnership or to have enough time for the children. For nothing, there is (almost) nothing in life!

Diabetes and Depression – Coping with Depression and Diabetes

Johannes Kruse Dejection, sadness, zero-buck mood: Many diabetics experience these feelings when their physical condition deteriorates, complications arise or limitations are experienced more clearly. Those affected are faced with the task of overcoming the challenge and adapting their lives to the limitations. We are talking about an adjustment or mourning process in which the person concerned comes to terms with the new situation. What can help in coping? A good relationship with his doctor, the support of friends and family, also the gathering of information, and the contingent of the individual strengths.

Many diabetics sooner or later develop depression: they feel depressed and powerless at the mercy of the situation; the mood can increase to pronounced feelings of helplessness, hopelessness, lack of drive, loss of interest, and strong self-esteem doubts. The future appears almost exclusively in shades of gray; you don't expect anything good – even if it looks quite different objectively.

Depression makes it difficult to deal with diabetes: some sufferers become increasingly indifferent and neglect their blood sugar control; others experience themselves as unreasonably helpless so that they develop strong fears of failing in therapy. To some, everything seems hopeless: "It doesn't help anyway... I can't do anything," are the complaints of a depressed patient. Due to the grey-tinted glasses, all upcoming tasks appear as unsolvable mountains: weight reduction, more movement – not to get everything out of the way. It is not surprising that depressed people often have poor blood sugar control. And at the same time, feelings of guilt that exceed the normal remorse are tormenting: some of those affected feel like failures, even if they do not fail objectively. They reproach themselves for not making the right effort, but the symptoms cannot be improved by more effort and by "pulling oneself together" – they are symptoms of a very stressful disease that needs to be treated.

The extent to which depression shapes the handling of the disease is shown by several current studies: They show that depressive diabetics adjust blood sugar levels worse than non-depressive diabetics and maintain weight reduction programs less often; they also smoke more often. Depression is also a risk factor for the development of coronary heart disease in diabetics, and it affects the quality of life of those affected much more than many other chronic physical diseases.

Breaking the circulation Depression and diabetes mellitus can mutually intensify.

Those affected can react to severe physical impairments with depression. On the other hand, the depressed mood makes it difficult for those affected to actively adjust to the disease and to control their blood sugar level. As a result, the quality of life decreases, and there is a risk that the experience will take a less favorable course; the cycle of depression and diabetes must be broken.

In the meantime, as already mentioned, there are several good therapeutic options for the treatment of depression: psychotherapy and/or drug treatment with antidepressants. If the problems of adaptation to the disease are in the foreground, the psychotherapeutic conversation is the method of choice; in moderate and severe depression, the method should be supplemented by therapy with modern antidepressants - meanwhile, some drugs are very poor in side effects.

Adequate treatment of depression not only improves the quality of life of affected patients - but also leads to improved metabolic control.

The Future of Diabetes Treatment: Is a Cure Possible? Yes, CLICK HERE

www.ingramcontent.com/pod-product-compliance
Lightning Source LLC
Chambersburg PA
CBHW070449220526
45466CB00004B/1787